Studies in Early Medicine 3

Series Editors: Sally Crawford and Christina Lee

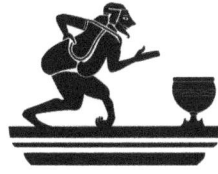

Social Dimensions of Medieval Disease and Disability

Edited by

Sally Crawford
Christina Lee

BAR International Series 2668
2014

Published in 2016 by
BAR Publishing, Oxford

BAR International Series 2668

Studies in Early Medicine 3
Social Dimensions of Medieval Disease and Disability

ISBN 978 1 4073 1310 8

BAR Publishing is the trading name of British Archaeological Reports (Oxford) Ltd.
British Archaeological Reports was first incorporated in 1974 to publish the BAR
Series, International and British. In 1992 Hadrian Books Ltd became part of the BAR
group. This volume was originally published by Archaeopress in conjunction with
British Archaeological Reports (Oxford) Ltd / Hadrian Books Ltd, the Series principal
publisher, in 2014. This present volume is published by BAR Publishing, 2016.

Printed in England

BAR
PUBLISHING

BAR titles are available from:

BAR Publishing
122 Banbury Rd, Oxford, OX2 7BP, UK
EMAIL   info@barpublishing.com
PHONE +44 (0)1865 310431
FAX   +44 (0)1865 316916
www.barpublishing.com

Foreword

Studies in Early Medicine is a peer-reviewed series designed to cover the growing discipline of the study of all aspects of disease, disability, health, medicine and society in the ancient and early medieval world, from prehistory to the Middle Ages. *Studies in Early Medicine* is interdisciplinary and multidisciplinary: papers from the fields of anthropology, archaeology, art, history, law, medicine and any other study relating to medicine, health and society in the pre-modern past in any geographical area are welcome.

Volumes will be devoted to a specific theme, interspersed by occasional general volumes, edited by a Guest Editor or Editors by agreement with the General Editors. Some volumes may arise out of conferences and workshops, but submissions of additional papers are welcome. We invite contributions on all aspects of early disease, medicine and healing. Future contributors may consult the associated website or the editors for further information: http://disease. nottingham.ac.uk/doku.php?do=show&id=journal_of_early_medicine.

General Editors

Dr Sally Crawford, Institute of Archaeology, 36 Beaumont Street, Oxford OX1 2PG

sally.crawford@arch.ox.ac.uk

Dr Christina Lee, School of English, University Park, Nottingham NG7 2RD

christina.lee@nottingham.ac.uk

Contents

Foreword 1

Contributors 3

Chapter 1
Introduction: social dimensions of medieval disease and disability 5
Sally Crawford

Chapter 2
The *unhal* and the semantics of Anglo Saxon disability 7
Fay Skevington

Chapter 3
Invisible enemies: the role of epidemics in the shaping of historical events in the early medieval period 15
Christina Lee

Chapter 4
The Madness of King Sigurðr: Narrating Insanity in an Old Norse Kings' Saga 29
Ármann Jakobsson

Chapter 5
'He was not an *idiota* from birth, nor is he now': false, temporary, and overturned charges of
mental incapacity in 14th-century England 37
Wendy Turner

Chapter 6
Disabling Masculinity: Manhood and Infertility in the High Middle Ages 47
Rachel Middlemass and Theresa Tyers

Chapter 7
Speechless: speech and hearing impairments as problem of medieval normative texts -
theological, natural-philosophical, legal 59
Irina Metzler

Chapter 8
Leprosy, Lepers and Leper-houses: between Human Law and God's Law (6th-15th centuries) 69
Damien Jeanne

Contributors

Dr Sally Crawford, The Institute of Archaeology, Oxford, UK
Sally.crawford@arch.ox.ac.uk

Professor Ármann Jakobsson, University of Iceland
armannja@hi.is

Dr Damien Jeanne, CRAHAM, Université de Caen, France
Damien.jeanne2@yahoo.fr

Dr Christina Lee, School of English, University of Nottingham
Christina.lee@nottingham.ac.uk

Rachel Middlemass, University College London
r.middlemass@ucl.ac.uk

Dr Irina Metzler, Wellcome Trust Research Fellow, MEMO Centre/Department of History, University of Swansea
research@irinametzler.org

Fay Skevington, Department of English Language and Literature, King's College London
Fay.skevington@kcl.ac.uk

Professor Wendy Turner, Department of History, Anthropology and Philosophy, Georgia Regents University, USA
wturner1@gru.edu

Theresa Tyers, University of Swansea
t.l.tyers@swansea.ac.uk

Chapter 1
Introduction: social dimensions of medieval disease and disability
Sally Crawford

The chronological and geographical focus of this volume is medieval northern Europe, from the 6th to the 15th centuries. In this volume, contributors examine the sometimes arbitrary social factors which resulted in people being deliberately, accidentally or temporarily categorised as disabled within their society, in ways that are peculiar to the medieval period. Health and disease are not static and unchanging; they are subject to cultural construction, manipulation and definition. Medieval ideas of healthy and unhealthy, as these papers show, were not necessarily - or even usually - comparable to modern approaches.

Each of the papers represented in this volume assesses social constructs of health and ill-health in different guises within the medieval period. How did medieval society define a 'normal' person in good health? And who were the arbiters of 'normal'? Doctors? Lawyers? Friends and neighbours? The church? If a given arbiter, in a position of authority, decided that an individual had broken the boundaries of 'normal' good health or 'ability', what were the social consequences for being 'unhealthy' or 'disabled'?

Fay Skevington introduces this theme with an important and insightful investigation into the ways in which Anglo-Saxon authors used the word *hal* and its antonym *unhal*, from which the modern words 'hale' and 'unhealthy' derive. Her intention, in this discussion, is to show the coverage of the Old English synonyms for 'unhealthy', and to allow us to develop a more nuanced idea of what Old English vocabulary allowed speakers to say and think about health. As she argues, understanding the meanings of a contemporary Anglo-Saxon term can serve to defamiliarize the concept of disability and unhook us from 'presentist assumptions' about medieval disease.

In her paper, Christina Lee assess the documentary and archaeological evidence for the role of disease as a *deus ex machina* in some of the major events of the early medieval period. Like Fay Skevington, she has to begin with terminology, because the literary sources for medieval disease and epidemics are notoriously unhelpful when it comes to identifying which particular kind of infectious disease a population was being affected by, as years of inconclusive scholarship on the thorny issue of the 'Justinian Plague' testify.

Ultimately, in terms of social, political and economic impact, it does not matter much whether the fatal epidemic was chickenpox or influenza. In terms of social change and population upheaval, the important issues are whether the proportion of the population killed by the infection was enough to destabilize society and cause economic breakdown, and whether the disease - through actual fatalities, or through a widespread perception that fatalities were likely - caused people to migrate away from the danger, or be drawn towards the opportunities presented by a vulnerable society with falling numbers and fragmenting infrastructures.

Lee surveys the surviving literature for evidence of significant epidemics as recounted by Old English, Frankish, Early Irish, Old Norse and Icelandic annals, saints' lives and sagas. In addition, she assesses the extent to which cemetery evidence, especially non-normative burial ritual, might offer an insight into the social dimension of epidemics across the early medieval period.

Lee's broad, synthetic view of the potential of early medieval documentary and archaeological evidence for understanding the impact of epidemics on populations in the widest sense, while Ármann Jakobsson focuses our attention on the consequences of one individual suffering from a malady. The extent to which a person is or is not affected by disease is a social construct. Social status, power relations and affective ties all require mediation and negotiation, and how the sufferer's identity and place in society is repositioned according to the perceptions of others about the meaning, cause, duration and impact of the affliction varies according to a complex interplay of personal and social factors, including status, gender, and age. These factors may have very little to do with biology and physiology. This cultural aspect of disease on social identity is exemplified in Jakobsson's study of the narrative reaction to a Norse king who suffered mental illness which caused him to behave in ways that could not be negotiated to fall within any societal 'norm', even for a king.

Jakobsson's Norse courtiers and chroniclers show compassion and sympathy for a good king who became mentally unstable. By contrast, Wendy Turner investigates the singularly self-interested and callous motivation of the 14th century accusers who tried to dispossess men and women of their property by levying false charges of idiocy against them.

In cases of disputed inheritance in later medieval England, it was the escheator's task to investigate the charge on behalf of the Crown. Escheators' records shed light on how the relative sanity or insanity of a person was tested and established in the late medieval period, and whether extended periods of lucidity could mitigate outbreaks of 'idiocy', or if temporary insanity - whether caused by disease or mental trauma - was enough to result in the confiscation of lands.

There was no simple test for medieval insanity - diagnosis depended heavily on opinion, reputation and behaviour. Male infertility might seem a more readily diagnosable medical condition, but as Rachel Middlemass and Theresa Tyres' paper shows, the subject was fraught with complications, and they emphasise the way in which understanding disease and disability from an historians' perspective requires a constant check on theory and terminology.

In particular, Middlemass and Tyers argue that male infertility falls into that grey area of diseases that only have a social impact and 'existence' in specific circumstances, and which may be completely 'transferred', in a social sense, onto another person who may be biologically and physiologically healthy. Effectively, a man does not suffer from sexual dysfunction until such time as he wants to have children and cannot. A man who chooses never to have children - a monk for example - might 'have' male infertility, but is in no way affected by the condition which is, therefore, neither problematic nor disabling. In social terms, such a person is entirely healthy.

If, on the other hand, a man wanted children but was infertile, the social and mental damage may be considerable, and so a condition which remains invisible and irrelevant to one person may be seriously disabling to another, with repercussions for his wider family, including, of course, his healthy wife, who may have the stigma of infertility transferred to her. Paradoxically, as the medieval records show, the healthy wife may be the focus of medical intervention, scrutiny and social stigma because of an untreated, uninvestigated and even unrecognised physiological abnormality in her husband.

The medieval legal implications of another kind of disability - deafness - are explored in Irina Metzler's survey of the congenital deaf-mute in Western Europe in the Middle Ages. Irina unpicks the complicated relationship between law, philosophy and theology as they affected the social, legal, ritual and economic lives of deaf-mutes, reminding the reader that the consequences of a disability depend on an interplay of ideology and social expectations. The social consequences of disability change over time according to prevailing theories and perceptions.

Perceptions and interpretations change over time - and this includes the prevailing theories historians use in their analyses of the past. How an historian 'reads' the past will be determined by a range of considerations, social, political and cultural. In this context, the volume concludes with a chapter by Damien Jeanne from the University of Caen, who analyzes the documentary sources for the social and religious attitudes to the medieval leper from c.500-c.1500. Jeanne places leprosy in an anthropological framework, a controversial and perhaps unfashionable methodology in the light of the scholarly conversation going on in the anglophone world today, but one which raises interesting points, and which will certainly encourage debate.

The majority of papers in this volume arose out of the sixth 'Disease and Disability in Medieval Europe' meeting at the University of Nottingham in 2011, organised by Dr Christina Lee: our thanks to the authors for bearing with us as this work was brought to publication. The papers in this volume were submitted to a peer review process. The editors would like to extend their sincere thanks to the referees for taking the time out of increasingly busy academic schedules, to offer thoughtful, rigorous and helpful comments.

Chapter 2
The *unhal* and the semantics of Anglo Saxon disability

Fay Skevington

Hit gelamp ða siððan æfter lytlum fyrste
on þæs cæseres dagum þe constantinus hatte
þæt sume menn sædon þa gesihþe his dehter
constantia gehaten seo wæs hæðen þagit
heo wæs swa þeah snotor and swyðe unhal
and on eallum limum egeslice wunda hæfde
þa ðohte heo þæt heo wolde wacian ane niht
æt agnes byrgene biddan hire hæle
Heo com þa þider þeah þe heo hæðen wære
and mid geleaf-fullum mode , to ðam mædene clypode
þe ða byrgene ahte þæt heo hyre hæle forgeafe
Heo wearð þa on slæpe and on swefne geseah
þa eadigan agnen þas word hire secgende
Ongin anrædlice ðu æðele constantia
and gelyf ðæt se hælend þe ge-hælen mæge
ðurh þone þu scealt underfon ðinra wunda hæle
þa awoc constantia and wæs swa ge-hæled
þæt on hire lice næs gesyne aht þæra sarra wunda
Heo ferde ða hal ham to hire fæder
and hine geblyssode and hire gebroðra
and ealle ða hired-menn for hire hæle blyssodon
and se hæðen-scipe wanode and godes geleafa weox

(Then it happened after a little while, in the days of the emperor who was called Constantine, that some men told the vision to his daughter called Constantia, who was still a heathen. She was, however, wise, and very unwell, and had awful wounds in all parts. Then she thought that she would wait one night at Agnes' tomb, to pray for her health. She came then came there, although she was heathen and with believing mind, called to the maiden who owned the tomb, that she would give her health. Then she drifted to sleep, and in a dream saw blessed Agnes, saying these words to her: 'Begin resolutely, noble Constantia, and believe that the Healer can heal you, through which you shall receive the healing of your wounds'. Then Constantia awoke, and was thus healed so that on her body nothing of the sore wounds was visible. Then she went home, whole, to her father, and gladdened him and her brothers, and all the household rejoiced because of her healing, and heathenism waned and God's faith waxed.) Ælfric's *Life of St Agnes* l.261-82.[1]

Although it depends on a Latin source, this healing narrative from Ælfric's late 10th-century life of St Agnes gives us some insight into the representation of physical impairment in Anglo-Saxon culture through the translator's selection of the text and lexical choices. Although Constantia's impairment is a key element of the narrative,

there is no description of her wounds other than to say they are *egeslic* ('awful') and the cause of the illness is not explained. This Old English text focuses on the social and spiritual implications of impairment, completely omitting causes or diagnoses of illness, unlike Latin versions in which she suffers from leprosy. In this text, Constantia's health status is correlated with her spiritual status. When she was a heathen, she was ill. Yet her wisdom (a typically Christian virtue) leads her towards faith, which enables her to be healed. The miracle also has a ripple effect, converting Constantia and the entire household, as *hæðen-scipe wanode and godes geleafa weox* ('heathenism waned and God's faith waxed'). In addition to her emerging faith, the narrative suggests that Constantia's physical proximity to holiness when she visits and sleeps in saint Agnes' tomb contributes to the healing miracle. The story teaches that holiness and illness cannot co-exist close to one another in the same textual space, as belief in Christ serves to cancel out physical impairment.

However, illness is not always negatively valued, even in Ælfric's *Lives of Saints*, which complicates any simple generalisations about the meanings ascribed to impairment by Anglo-Saxon textual culture. To take another example, St Martin seems to revel in his illness:

Eft ða he ham wolde þa wearð he ge-untrumod
and sæde his gebroðrum þæt he sceolde forð-faren
Þa wurdon hi ealle ge-unrotsode swiþe
and mid micelre heofunge hine befrinan
Eala þu fæder hwi forlætst þu us ...
þa wearð se halga wer mid þysum wordum astyrod
and clypode mid wope and cwæð to his drihtne
Drihten min hælend gif ic nyd-behefe eom
git þinum folce ne for-sace ic na
gyt to swincene gewurðe þin willa
Ne ic ne beladige mine ateorigendlican ylde
ic þine þenunga est-ful gefylde under þinum tacnum
ic campige swa lange swa þu sylf hætst
He lag þa swa forþ ane feawa daga
mid fefore gewæht þurh-wunigende on ge-bedum
on stiþre hæran licgende mid axum bestreowod
Þa bædon þa gebroðra þæt hi his bæd moston
mid waccre strewunge huru under-lecgan
Þa cwæð se halga wer to þam wependum gebroðrum
Ne gedafnað cristenum menn buton þæt he on duste swelte
gif ic eow oþre bysne selle þonne syngie ic
He ne let na of gebedum his un-oferswiððan gast
ac he æfre openum eagum and up-ahafenum handum
his gebeda ne geswac Þa woldon þa preostas
þæt he lage on oþre sidan and ge-lihte hine swa
þa cwæð se halga eft Geþafiað ic bidde
þæt ic heofonan sceawige swiðor þonne eorðan

[1] Skeat 1966.

(Afterwards, when he wished to return home, he became ill and said to his brothers that he would die. Then they were all very saddened and with great lamentation asked him 'Alas, why do you forsake us father...' Then the holy man was moved by these words and called with weeping, and said to his Lord, 'Lord my Healer, if I am still necessary to your people, I will nor give up work to honour your will, nor plead the excuse of my failing age. Devout, I fulfilled your service. Under your sign I fight so long as you yourself command'. He then lay thus for a few days longer, weakened with fever, continuing in prayers, lying on stiff haircloth strewn with ashes. Then the brothers asked that they might at least underlay his bed with more yielding bedding.

Then the holy man said to the weeping brothers 'It does not befit a Christian man but that he dies in the dust. If I gave you another example, then I would sin'. He did not release his unconquered spirit from prayers, but with ever open eyes and raised up hands, he did not cease his prayers. Then the priests wished that he would lie on the other side, and thus rest himself. Then the saint said 'I ask, allow me to look on heaven rather than the earth'.) Ælfric's *Life of St Martin, Bishop and Confessor*, l.1330-4, 1341-63.[2]

There are some similarities in the way that impairment is described in these examples of Agnes and Martin. As in the Life of St Agnes, there is no mention of the cause of Martin's illness; he simply *ge-untrumod* ('becomes ill') and in both narratives, those close to the impaired individual see their condition as undesirable. This is demonstrated by the solicitude of Martin's brethren in attempting to lessen his suffering and in the joyful reaction of Constantia's family when she is cured. According to general consensus of supporting characters, impairment is negatively valued.

However, Martin the Archbishop and Saint re-inscribes the meaning of his illness as positive; indeed, as an intrinsically holy state befitting a Christian. He lies on hair cloth, strewn with ashes, refusing softer bedding or to be turned onto his side, and continues to pray, eventually managing to dispose of a devil before he dies. The opportunities for holiness provided by impairment are therefore two-fold. Firstly, Martin demonstrates the strength of his dedication to his Christian vocation, continuing to serve despite the difficulties caused by his illness. Secondly, in his refusal to accept interventions to lessen his suffering, he demonstrates his humility, and his ability to transcend his physical condition in favour of his spiritual existence. For Martin, the implication is that to ameliorate the symptoms of disease would be to decrease in holiness.

These contrasting deployments of disease demonstrate the difficulties of making generalisations about the meanings that Anglo-Saxon culture ascribes to physical impairment. But if understanding the meanings of disease and disability in Anglo-Saxon culture is challenging, this is not helped by the difficulties of present day definitions and nomenclature. That what constitutes disability is so contentious and fraught with concerns of miscategorisation emphasises how fundamental the control, regulation and categorisation of bodies is to how we make sense of the world. As Mary Douglas would argue, the body is the primary source of metaphor and semiotics.[3]

In discussing the conditions of Martin and Constantia, for example, I have used 'illness' and 'impairment' interchangeably. Indeed, it is hard to delineate clearly the boundaries between concepts of illness, disability, and disease in modern discourse. In the UK, the legal meaning of disability is given by the Equalities Act 2010, which defines a person with a disability as a person who has (or has had) a physical or mental impairment which has a substantial and long-term (over 12 months) adverse effect on the individual's ability to carry out normal day-to-day activities. This encompasses long-term physical and mental illnesses, in addition to conditions caused by accidents or congenital disabilities. But the blurring of the boundary between disability and disease can be problematic and even uncomfortable for people who do or do not identify as disabled. Indeed, the language of disability is so fraught that the UK government Office for Disability Issues has a prescriptive guide to acceptable language.[4] However, even this guide seems to contradict itself in some places. For example, it suggests that we should '[u]se 'disabled people' as the collective term... Avoid medical labels which tend to reinforce stereotypes'. However, the very next suggestion is:

> Don't refer solely to 'disabled people' ... many people who need disability benefits and services do not identify with this term. 'People with health conditions or impairments' is another common descriptor.

Thus the advice is rather conflicted: 'disabled people' is to be used as the collective term, but not all the time, and medical labels should be avoided, although 'people with health conditions' is appropriate.

Whilst these modern nuances may be confusing, I would argue that a lack of distinction between illness and disability is appropriate when discussing Anglo-Saxon culture. As the descriptions of Constantia's and Martin's illnesses demonstrate, there is little focus on establishing the type of illness, or its cause. Old English medical texts such as the *Leechbook* do occasionally supply causes for the diseases for which cures are given, worms and elves being amongst the most memorable, which only serves as a reminder of the fundamentally different paradigm in which Anglo-Saxon perceptions of disease were explored. Furthermore,

---

[2]Skeat 1966. A similar narrative occurs in the *Blickling Homily* (Kelly 2003, 146-56).

[3]Douglas 1970.
[4]Issues 2010, http://odi.dwp.gov.uk/inclusive-communications/representation/language.php accessed 30/04/2011.

many conditions which would not be seen as long term today, such as a broken leg, could have been permanently disabling for an Anglo-Saxon individual. Distinctions between illness and disability in Anglo-Saxon literature therefore risk imposing a modern medical taxonomy of causality and curability on a discursive artefact of a culture which would not recognise such a categorisation.

To understand medieval cultural interpretations of disability, therefore, we need to interrogate our own theoretical concepts of disability in addition to understanding which conditions we classify as a disability. Modern disability studies have explored several models of disability. The medical model, in which disabilities are aberrations which must be cured, was challenged by disability activists in the 1970s, who developed the social model of disability. Under the social model of disability, disability and impairment are distinguished, whereby impairment describes the actual physical condition of a body, and disability describes the social reception of that body. As a result of impairments, people are oppressed and thus disabled by society.

Given that within a social model, disability can be seen as socially constructed as opposed to a physical fact, Irina Metzler questions whether medieval impaired people were actually socially oppressed on the basis of their impairment.[5] For medieval disability, Edward Wheatley suggests that a religious model is appropriate, analogous to the medical model, but where the Church controls the meaning of disability and seeks to remedy the problem of the disabled person through salvation and healing.[6] However, without denying the power of the medieval Church in ascribing meaning to bodies, we do need to be wary of implying that the category of disabled is somehow transhistorical and universal, even though the institutions which regulate disability change. Paul Abberly, for example, laments the absence of 'significant recognition of the historical specificity of the experience of disability'.[7] Robert McRuer explores the way that disability is created by capitalism, and asserts that 'being able-bodied means being capable of the normal physical exertions required in a particular system of labor'.[8] Vic Finkelstein, working in disability studies in the 1970s and 80s, also linked disability and capitalism, suggesting three phases in the development of disability.[9] Phase 1, defined by the feudal system and small scale industry and agriculture, was a period during which disabled people were not discriminated against and were able to make a contribution. Phase 2 covers the industrial revolution, in which disabled people were excluded and suffered discrimination. Phase 3, into which we are entering, will be characterized by independent living for disabled people thanks to technological developments. Such idealisation of the medieval period as

a permissive time before discrimination can be compared to Foucault's ideas about medieval sexuality.[10] Whilst these categorisations optimistically place the medieval period in an idealised golden age where oppression on the grounds of impairment or sexuality did not exist *per se*, it does highlight the cultural and historical specificity of the production of disability.

Josh Eyler, in his introduction to *Disability in the Middle Ages*, suggests that a cultural model, based on the work of Mitchell and Snyder, is appropriate for discussing medieval disability.[11] He argues that both social conditions and corporeality (or impairment) produce the effects of disability. According to Eyler: 'this less divisive model allows us to take into account the entire spectrum of experiences for people with disabilities and does not force us to focus on constructed perceptions of disability at the expense of real, bodily phenomena'.[12]

The theoretical approaches to medieval disability explored so far are dependent on a distinction between impairment and disability, but recent work has begun to investigate the problematic nature of this impairment/disability split. Tom Shakespeare and Nicholas Watson, for example, argue that just as Judith Butler posits the social constructedness of sex, impairment (as opposed to socially defined disability) is also socially constructed. They argue that how people are treated depends on not only how disabling (or not) a society is to impaired people, but also on what constitutes impairment within that society. Everyone is impaired, to a greater or lesser degree: society has adapted to cater for some impairments, but not others: 'While all living beings are impaired - that is, frail, limited, vulnerable, mortal - we are not all oppressed on the basis of this impairment and illness'.[13]

Although it is only disability that is traditionally seen as having a social dimension, it becomes clear that what constitutes impairment is also dependent on social conditions. For example, in a largely illiterate society, an Anglo-Saxon labourer would have been unlikely to have been limited by dyslexia. Ideas about impairment, like those about disability, are never neutral, but are always already imbued with cultural judgments.

If finding ways of defining, talking and thinking about disability in our own culture is hard, then it is hardly surprising that it is challenging to develop a critical language to explore these issues in the culture of over one thousand years ago. If both impairment and disability are culturally or socially constructed, then we need to acknowledge the historical specificity of both impairment and disability in different cultures. We have to be aware that the concept of 'medieval disability' is to some extent a projection of our own frameworks of meaning, imposing

---

[5] Metzler 2006.
[6] Wheatley 2010, 10-9.
[7] Abberly 1987, 6.
[8] McRuer 2006, 91-92.
[9] Finkelstein 1980.

[10] Foucault 1978.
[11] Eyler 2010; Snyder and Mitchell 2006; Mitchell and Snyder 2000.
[12] Eyler 2010, 6.
[13] Shakespeare and Watson 2001, 25.

our own category of 'disabled' on the past, in the same way that the concept of medieval sexuality can be seen as a construction.[14]

Given the difficulty of applying these socially constructed meanings of illness, disease and impairment to a chronologically distant society, I would like instead to propose the use of an Old English term, which may help us to extricate ourselves from the semantic and political tangles of disability vocabulary. *Unhal* is a cognate of Modern English 'unhealthy', and the antonym of *hal,* which reaches us in Modern English as 'whole' and 'hale'. However, the Old English meaning of *unhal* covers more than simply 'unhealthy'. Given that the Toronto Dictionary of Old English has yet to reach 'u', let alone 'h', we have to refer to Bosworth and Toller, who define '*un-hál*; adj. In bad health, sick, weak, infirm, unhealthy, unsound'.[15]

Old English cognates include:

> *un-hælþ*; bad health, sickness, weakness, infirmity

> *un-hælu*; I. bad health, disease, sickness, infirmity; II. misfortune, mishap .

Unhælþ and *unhælu* occur largely as nominal forms, whereas *unhal* is usually adjectival, albeit with instances of functional shift where it occurs as a noun (i.e. 'the sick'). The following extract from the *Life of St Margaret* in MS Corpus Christi College Cambridge 303, lists some of the conditions which are classified as *unhal*'

> *þæt innan heora husum nan* unhal *cild sy geboren, ne crypol, ne dumb, ne deaf, ne blind, ne ungewittes.*

> (That in their house no *unwhole* child be born, neither cripple nor dumb, nor deaf, nor blind, nor mad).[16]

This demonstrates that the conditions covered by *unhal* seem largely similar to present day 'disability' (note that Elaine Treharne translates *unhal* in this text as 'disabled'[17]). The Latin Life and the other Old English text (found in Cotton Tiberius A. iii.) list the conditions which can be avoided by ownership of the text of Margaret's life, but these texts do not group these impairments into a single category as MS CCCC 303 does.[18] This Anglo-Saxon text therefore adds the concept of the *unhal* or the disabled as a specifically recognised category. Indeed, its appearance in Cnut's and Æthelred's law codes, and in the penitential text, the *Old English Handbook,* suggests that being *unhal* was a status or condition recognised before secular and religious authorities.[19] This extract from the *Life of St Margaret* also suggests the cultural undesirability of the

unhal, in that it is something to be avoided through St Margaret's intercession.

In modern idiom, the conditions covered in the prayer of St Margaret fall squarely within the remit of a discourse of impairment. However, *hal,* from which *unhal* is derived, and its cognates show a moral dimension:

> *hál*; whole, hale, well, in good health, sound, safe, without fraud, honest

> *hælþ*; health, healing, cure

> *hælu*; health, safety, salvation

Thus it is clear that whilst, according to Bosworth and Toller, *unhal* covers the semantic field of sickness, injury and disability, its antonym *hal* has a strong moral component, suggesting that *unhal* is not a morally neutral term. The *Oxford English Dictionary,* under the form *unhal* of 'unwhole, a' gives the following definitions for occurrences in Old English:

a. Not in good health; unsound, unhealthy; diseased, infirm, sick...

b. Spiritually or morally unsound.

Additionally, under 'unheal', where the Old English form is *unhæl* (-o/-u), the *OED* defines 'Want of health or soundness; infirmity, trouble, misfortune'. The moral dimension of *unhal* and its cognates is evidenced by its usage in Old English. For example, *unhal* is particularly associated with over indulgence, and by extension, sin, as in this example from Ælfric's Old English version of *De Duodecim Abusivis*: *Se oferlyfa on æte & on wæte deð þone man unhalne & his sawle gode læðetteð swa swa ure drihten on his godspelle cwæð*.[20] (The over enjoyment of food and drink makes a man[21] unwell/unwholesome and god scorns his soul, just as our lord says in his gospel.)

In these and similar definitions, there is a repeated connection to food, which is hardly surprising given its significance as a point of contact between physical and spiritual wellbeing.[22] For example a Wulfstanian homily asserts: *Oferfyll bið þære sawle feond and þæs lichaman unhæl* ('Overfullness is the enemy of the soul and the sickness of the body')[23] while the Old English Dicts of Cato tells us that *Gif ðu wylle hal beon, drinc ðe gedæftlice; ælc oferfyll & ælc idel fett unhælo.*[24]

For a Vercelli homilist, specific types of overindulgence and ill health are gendered. For women *unhal* is not the

[14] See for example Lochrie, McCracken *et al.* 1997.
[15] Bosworth, Toller and Campbell 1972.
[16] Clayton and Magennis 1994, 168.
[17] Treharne 2004, 271.
[18] Clayton and Magennis 1994.
[19] Liebermann 1898; Fowler 1965, 20; Frantzen 2011.

[20] Morris 1868, 296.
[21] Old English *mann* had the general meaning of 'person', and while for Anglo-Saxons the prototypical person was doubtless male, the semantic range of *mann* was wider, cf, Fell 2002, 201-7.
[22] *cf.* Walker Bynum 1987.
[23] Napier 1883, 242.
[24] 1.60; Cox 1972.

consequence of over-eating, but of the adornment and washing of the body:

> Eawla, wif, to hwan wenest ðu þines lichoman hæle <geican> mid smyringe & oftþweale & oðrum liðnessum? Of ðam cymeð unhælo, nals mægen.

> (Oh, woman, why do you hope to augment your healthy body with anointment and frequent washing and other indulgences? From this comes unwholesomeness, not at all strength).[25]

In yet another homily, the association of *unhæl* with sin is illustrated as *unhæl* is an inherent property of hell:

> *Ac eac hit is mid wyrmum afylled and mid wean and mid wræcsiðan, þær næfre leoht ne leomað. ac þær bið þeostru beþrycced and hungor and þurst and heto and yldo and unhælo and wanung and granung and toða grisbitung.*

> (But it is also filled with worms, and with pain and exile, where light never shines. But there is pressing darkness, and hunger and thirst and hate and age and illness and moaning and groaning and toothgrinding).[26]

Unhal, however, is not only associated with infirmity (although that is the most common meaning), but can also be associated with an unwholesome size or strength:

> *Swa is eac on lichaman se læssa man betere, swa swa Zacheus wæs, mid gesundfulnysse, þonne se unhala beo and hæbbe on his wæstme Golian mycelnysse, þæs gramlican entes.*

> (Thus in the same way in the body, the lesser, healthy man is better, just as Zacheus was, than to be unwholesome and have the Goliath-like greatness of stature of the hostile giant). *Homily for the Nativity of the Blessed Virgin Mary.*[27]

Unhal and *unhælu* are predominantly used in prose, although *unhal* occurs twice in poetry, both times in the metrical psalms. *Unhælu* too occurs twice in verse, once in the *Seasons for Fasting*, and once in *Beowulf*. Bosworth and Toller gloss *Beowulf*'s *unhælo* in line 120 as the single instance of a secondary meaning for *unhælu*, meaning misfortune or mishap. However, more recently the reference to Grendel as *wiht unhælo* (l.120) has been translated as 'God-cursed brute', by Heaney.[28] This, and similar translations, are presumably posited on translating *unhælu* as the direct opposite of *hælu*, 'salvation', although it can just as easily mean 'health'.[29] However, given that

wiht unhælo is followed by *grim ond graédig*, one could equally translate this as referring to the unwholesomeness resulting from Grendel's overindulgent consumption of human flesh, or indeed, to his uncanny size and strength, similar to the reference to *gramlican entes* in the extract from the Marian homily quoted above.

As these examples indicate, it is hard to be clear which exact sense of *unhal* or *unhælu* is being used on many occasions; spiritual degeneracy or physical or mental impairment seem almost interchangeable. If there is a permeable boundary between *unhæl* and *unhælþ*, which both have a strong moral component, and between them both and *unhal*, there is also overlap with *un-hálig*; (adj. 'Unholy'), and related words. Given the inherent variability of Anglo-Saxon spellings, we might question the applicability of a strict verbal taxonomy for this semantic cluster.[30]

Unhal can mean not yet saved or cured; unwholesome, sick, not whole, weak or not honest/good. Its literal meaning, 'un-whole', demonstrates the underlying assumption of deviation from a bodily ideal. Even the morphological underpinnings of the terms can be revealing. *Unhal* suggests subjects and bodies come into being through processes of completion or salvation, and remind us of the importance of fragmentation as a cultural motif.[31] We are also freed of the associations of 'disability' in a capitalist paradigm of production, where bodies and subjects are made viable by what they can do or make. Whilst scholars looking for evidence of direct oppression of medieval impaired people may not find a great deal, the confusion of moral and physical impairment in the definition of *unhal* suggests oppression: to label an individual sinful on account of impairment is an inherently disabling judgement. *Unhal* therefore denotes impairment in addition to demonstrating the oppression (or disabling) by society of the impaired body including through moral judgements made about those bodies.

Unhal could describe both a condition caused by sin and a condition to be cured by healing, both sickness and disability, both deformation and weakness and both a mental and a physical condition. Positively valued impairments, such as those incurred through martyrdom, however, are excluded from these terms. In practice, these prestige impairments were largely accessible only to the religious elite, and frequently only to a historical and

---

[25] *Vercelli Homily VII*, l. 72-5 (Scragg 1992. See also Zacher 2009, 98-150).

[26] *Wednesday in Rogationtide* l.62-4 (Bazire and Cross 1982).

[27] Assmann 1889.

[28] Heaney 1999.

[29] *Cf* Bradley 1995.

[30] The *Thesaurus of Old English* has entries for *unhal* and related words. However, these high level categorisations do not give us a great deal of insight into any specific nuances for this cluster of words. Instead, it appears that the these terms have similarly variable meanings:

Hæl(u): Salvation, redemption; Sound physical condition.

Hælu: Mental/spiritual health; Healing, curing.

Hælþ: Mental/spiritual health; Healing, curing; Salvation, redemption.

Hal: Sound Physical condition - Healthy; Sound Mind - In one's right mind, sane - (Of mind) sane, sound; Uninjured, unhurt, unharmed - Purity, moral cleaness - Pure, whole, pure of heart.

Unhal: Disease, infirmity, sickness- Sick, ill, diseased; Animal diseases - Unsound

(Roberts, Kay et al 2000).

[31] *cf.* Walker Bynum 1991.

therefore disembodied subset of this community (although one could argue that such prestige impairments are made more accessible to lived experience in later periods with the rise of anchoritic spirituality as evidenced, for example, by *Ancrene Wisse*).[32] The sick that Lucy, Agnes, and Swithun in the Old English versions of their *Lives* cure are described as *unhal* from a variety of causes and symptoms. But although saints themselves may be wounded, struck down, or weak, they are never described as *unhal*: holiness can overcome *unhal*, but the holy can never be *unhal*. This re-enforces the case for the importance of the shared etymology of *hal* and *halig*.

To return to the two examples from Ælfric's lives of Saints, we see that Constantia is *unhal*, whereas Martin is *untrum*. Constantia's unwholeness is not limited to her physical status. She was 'as yet a heathen', the description of her as *unhal* also hinting at her spiritually incomplete status. Martin's illness is merely a physical condition, which does not affect his spiritual status, other than to enhance it. Martin and Constantia follow two different biblical archetypes which give contrasting meanings to impairment. Martin follows Christ's example, welcoming impairment and suffering for his flock in a gesture of self sacrifice. This 'holy suffering' trope is distinct from Constantia's experience of impairment. Instead, she moves from a spiritually deprived state, seeking cure for her physical illness, and is cured by Christ and her new-found faith. This 'sick in need of healing' model can be seen to be based on biblical examples such as Christ's healing of the blind man.

David Mitchell and Sharon Snyder use the idea of 'narrative prosthesis' to refer to both the use of the disabled body as a kind of narrative 'crutch', where the exceptional body is a point of departure, and the subsequent cover-up (through cure, erasure or punishment) of the disabled body to restore the hegemonic 'able-bodied' order.[33] Following this concept of 'narrative prosthesis', *unhal* can be seen as analogous to a plot device which ultimately requires resolution; the concept of the *unhal*, by its very nature, needs to be made whole. However, it is interesting and striking that not all impairment in Anglo-Saxon literature is follows the narrative prosthesis trope, but, for example can be an intensifier of and route to holiness. In these instances, impairment is more likely to be referred to as *untrumnesse* or another neutrally valued term.

Unhal therefore describes the cultural location of stigmatised disability in Anglo-Saxon England, encapsulating impairments arising through disease, injury or congenital condition. It also reflects the ambiguous reception of these conditions, where a lack of physical or sensory 'wholeness' can be associated with, and subject to judgements about a lack of spiritual wholeness.[34] But similarities between the function of modern disability and Anglo-Saxon *unhal* should not be seen as licence to continue using modern models of disability: universalising narratives of disability can obscure variations of meaning within a culture, let alone across cultures.

Carelessly applying a cultural model of disability which elides impairment and disability could suggest that disabled people face similar cultural difficulties in whichever society they exist. Thus adopting 'disability' as a universal term could therefore be seen to reverse the enabling possibilities of the social model of disability. *Unhal* is a culturally specific term for one particular cultural reception of impairment, and using it acknowledges the existence of other interpretations and productions of impairment, both synchronically and diachronically. Using *unhal* can therefore acknowledge the oppression of some impaired Anglo-Saxon individuals, without impinging on the aims of the social model adopted in order to further disability activism. As the meaning of *unhal* is specific, it does not foreclose neutral or more positive cultural meanings in other societies or for other productions of impairment in Anglo-Saxon society. It is, of course, worth remembering that by their nature, impairments which were neutrally valued and not stigmatised are unlikely to be significantly represented in extant cultural evidence. In literature, we only see the cultural traces of disability; we can never truly excavate the 'real' impairment, if we accept this concept at all.

I'd like to make clear that I do not intend to argue that *unhal* is the most popular term for this semantic field, nor that it is the direct equivalent of our modern term 'disabled': at least one other candidate might be *untrum*, as we have seen. Instead I would like to suggest using this term as a way of, if not extricating ourselves from, then at least loosening our ties to 'presentist assumptions' as Lochrie, when talking about medieval sexuality, calls them. Using a contemporary Anglo-Saxon term can serve to defamiliarise the concept of disability and problematise the presumed universality of disability. Talking about disease, disability, weakness, or sickness will always be imbued with modern, often medical, connotations. Rather, the points of contact and divergence between *unhal* and disability allows us to explore the cultural construction of, and responses to, impairment.

---

[32] See also royal impairments: Tovey 2010.
[33] Mitchell and Snyder 2000, 49.

[34] We could perhaps draw parallels between *unhal* and 'sick', which can both mean illness and debility, as well as meaning wrong or repulsive. See McRuer for discussion and reclamation of the word 'sick', particularly his discussion of 'Bob Flanagan's Sick' (McRuer 2006).

Bibliography

Abberly, P. 1987. 'The concept of oppression and the development of a social theory of disability'. *Disability and Handicap in Society*, **2**, 5-19.

Assmann, B. and Grein, C.W.(eds) 1889. *Angelsèachsische Homilien und Heiligenleben*. Kassel.

Bazire, J. and Cross, J.E. (eds) 1982. *Eleven Old English Rogationtide homilies*. Toronto Old English series; 7. Toronto: University of Toronto Press.

Bosworth, J., Toller, T.N. and Campbell, A. 1972. *An Anglo-Saxon dictionary, based on the manuscript collections of Joseph Bosworth: Enlarged Addenda and Corrigenda*. Oxford: Clarendon Press.

Bradley, S.A.J., (ed) 1995. *Anglo-Saxon poetry*. London: Everyman.

Clayton, M. and Magennis, H. (eds) 1994. *The Old English lives of St. Margaret*. Cambridge: Cambridge University Press.

Cox, R.S. 1972. 'The Old English Dicts of Cato'. *Anglia*, **90**, 1-42.

Douglas, M.M. 1970. *Natural Symbols: Explorations in Cosmology*, London: Routledge.

Eyler, J. 2010. 'Introduction: breaking boundaries, building bridges', in J. Eyler (ed) *Disability in the Middle Ages: Reconsiderations and Reverberations*, 1-10. Surrey: Ashgate.

Fell, C.E., 2002. 'Words and women in Anglo-Saxon England', in C. Hough and K.A. Lowe (eds), *'Lastworda Betst': Essays in Memory of Christine E. Fell with her Unpublished Writings*, 198-215. Donington: Tyas.

Finkelstein, V. 1980. *Attitudes and Disabled People: Issues for Discussion*. Michigan: The University of Michigan Press.

Foucault, M. (Hurley, R. trans.) 1978. *The history of sexuality: Volume 1: An Introduction*, London: Pantheon Books.

Fowler, R. 1965. 'A Late Old English Handbook for the use of a confessor'. *Anglia - Zeitschrift fur englishe Philologie*, **83**, 1-34.

Frantzen, A. 2011. *The Anglo-Saxon Penitentials: a Cultural Database*: http://www.anglo-saxon.net/penance/

Heaney, S. 1999. *Beowulf*, London: Faber and Faber.

Issues, O.F.D. 2010. *Language*. Retrieved 30/04, 2011, from http://odi.dwp.gov.uk/inclusive-communications/representation/language.php

Kelly, R.J. (ed. and trans.)2003. *The Blickling Homilies*, London: Continuum.

Liebermann, F. 1898. *Die Gesetze der Angelsachsen*. Halle: Max Steinmeyer.

Lochrie, K., McCracken, P. and Schultz, J.A. (eds) 1997. *Constructing Medieval Sexuality*, Minneapolis: University of Minnesota Press.

McRuer, R. 2006. *Crip Theory: Cultural Signs of Queerness and Disability*, New York: New York University Press.

Metzler, I. 2006. *Disability in Medieval Europe: Thinking about Physical Impairment during the High Middle Ages, c.1100-1400*, London: Routledge.

Mitchell, D.T. and Snyder, S.L. 2000. *Narrative Prosthesis: Disability and the Dependencies of Discourse*, Ann Arbor: University of Michigan Press.

Morris, R., (ed.) 1868. *Old English Homilies and Homiletic Treatises: 1st series*, Oxford: Clarendon Press.

Napier, A.S., (ed) 1883. *Sammlung der ihm zugeschriebenen Homilien 4: Wulfstan*, Berlin: Wiedmann.

Roberts, J.A., Kay, C. and Grundy, L. (eds) 2000. *A Thesaurus of Old English: Volume 1*, Amsterdam: Rodopi.

Scragg, D.G. (ed.) 1992. *The Vercelli Homilies and Related Texts*, Oxford.

Shakespeare, T. and Watson, N. 2001. 'The social model of disability: an outdated ideology?', in S.N. Barnartt and B.M. Altman (eds), *Exploring Theories and Expanding Methodologies: Where we are and Where we need to go*, 9-28. London: Emerald Group Publishing Limited.

Skeat, W.W. (ed.) (1881, repr. 1966). *Aelfric's Lives of Saints: Being a Set of Sermons on Saints' Days Formerly Observed by the English Church*, 2 Volumes, London: EETS.

Snyder, S.L. and Mitchell, D.T. 2006. *Cultural Locations of Disability*, Chicago: University of Chicago Press.

Tovey, B. 2010. 'Kingly impairments in Anglo-Saxon literature: God's curse and God's blessing', in J. Eyler (ed), *Disability in the Middle Ages: Reconsiderations and Reverberations*. 135-48. Surrey: Ashgate.

Treharne, E.M. (ed) 2004. *Old and Middle English c.890-c.1400: an anthology*, Oxford: Blackwell.

Walker Bynum, C. 1987. *Holy Feast and Holy Fast: the Religious Significance of Food to Medieval Women*, Berkeley and Los Angeles: University of California Press.

Walker Bynum, C. 1991. *Fragmentation and Redemption: Essays on Gender and the Human Body in Medieval Religion*, New York: Zone Press.

Wheatley, E. 2010. *Stumbling Blocks Before the Blind: Medieval Constructions of a Disability*, Ann Arbor: University of Michigan Press.

Zacher, S. 2009. 'The source of Vercelli VII: an address to women', in A. Orchard and S. Zacher (eds), *New readings in the Vercelli book*, 98-150. Toronto: University of Toronto Press.

Chapter 3
Invisible enemies: the role of epidemics in the shaping of historical events in the early medieval period

Christina Lee

Introduction

In this chapter I wish to sketch what is known about outbreaks of infectious disease in northern Europe - linguistic, textual and material - and consider the impact that these events may have had on their societies. The chapter is borne out of an ongoing interest in the Viking migrations, which saw a shift from small bands going on seasonal raids in the 8th century to a large-scale migration in the 9th. The Viking Age saw the greatest expansion of Scandinavian cultural influence in history, and among the reasons put forward for this expansion - technical ability, demographic necessity or ideological inevitability,[1] the role that infectious disease may have played in both the expansion and the decline of Viking and Norse influence across the North Atlantic has not been fully examined. The chapter considers potential sources of information for epidemics in early medieval Britain and Ireland, and considers if disease may have accelerated changes which altered the political and economic landscape of early medieval Britain and Ireland, to a point which eventually allowed for the colonisation of Anglo-Saxon, Scottish and Irish regions by Scandinavians, areas from which many settlers to the new lands across the Atlantic were drawn. The chapter will consider the type of disease that may be lurking behind the ubiquitous term 'plague', and consider the role that disease played in the beginning and the end of the Viking diaspora expansion across the North Atlantic.

The possibility that a wide-spread pandemic, thought to be a northern expansion of the Justinian Plague (AD 540-2), affected Britain and Ireland in the 8th century has been discussed by a number of scholars in the past,[2] but has been largely ignored by most scholars who study the fundamental changes affecting Middle Anglo-Saxon England. The reason why so little attention may have been paid to a potential epidemic and its social and economic fallout lies in the fact that until very recently it was generally accepted that the Black Death pandemic of the 14th century was the first of its kind in Europe. All other reported outbreaks of disease were not seen as connected, but rather as localised calamities. Additionally, the medieval historians who could have told us about it, have often remarkably little interest in the health of their contemporaries, in the same way as they do not often talk about floods, earthquakes or other natural phenomena. When they do talk about disease, it is often in images and metaphors which are heavily reliant on traditions inherited from classical antiquity.[3] Such conventions, and the incomplete and obscure nature of much of early medieval documentation, has led to the oversight of the study of infectious disease.

Plague? What plague?

One of the most difficult aspects of examining past diseases is that there is no consensus on the nature, severity or even existence of epidemics among scholars. Even when sickness is explicitly mentioned in early medieval sources, the vocabulary used to describe it is often quite vague. The term that is generally used by medieval writers for any kind of epidemic is Latin *pestilentia*, 'pestilence'. This word appears to cover a multitude of different diseases, but we should note that writers who use the vernacular often differentiate their vocabulary in order to distinguish between diseases, or at least to avoid repetition. The relationship between the various words used for infectious diseases is still waiting for a detailed study of chronological and regional semantic variations, but I will introduce briefly the main terms used for infectious disease.

Most of our knowledge of outbreaks to date still comes from literary texts, and scholars are often wary of the written word. However, even though texts should be read with caution, it is worth noting that although disease and calamity are only sporadically mentioned in historical sources, let alone literature, when they are mentioned this has significance for the writer and audience. Illness may be a convenient plot device for getting rid of unpopular rulers, such as Theudebald in Gregory of Tour's *History of the Franks*[4] or Harthacnut's demise in 1041 in the E-version of the *Anglo-Saxon Chronicle*,[5] where it may fulfil a didactic function, but there are cases, as I will show, where authors are telling us about outbreaks and consequences.

Most scholars who argued that the plague ravaged Europe prior to the 14th century have based their arguments largely on written sources. They have pointed out that there are similarities between descriptions of the Justinian Plague and later outbreaks. One of the most descriptive sources for the Justinian Plague is by the contemporary Byzantine author Procopius in his *History of the Wars:*

> During these times there was a pestilence, by which the whole human race came near to being annihilated. [...] For it left neither island nor cave nor mountain ridge which had human inhabitation and it passed by any land, either not affecting the men there or touching them in different fashion, still at a later time

---

[1] Barrett 2008.
[2] Creighton 1891; Bonser 1963; Maddicot 2007; Dooley 2007.
[3] Slack 1992, 9.
[4] Krusch and Levison 1961, 141.
[5] Irvine 2004, 77.

it came back; then those who dwelt round this land, whom formerly it had afflicted most sorely, it did not touch at all.

Procopius relates that it would kill equal numbers of those who had previously been unaffected. He continues that the disease always ran from the coast inland. Historians and palaeopathologists have been most interested in the description of the disease which follows this section:

> But with the majority it came about that they were seized by the disease without becoming aware of what was coming [...] They had a sudden fever [...]. And the body showed no change from its previous colour, nor was it hot as might be expected when attacked by a fever, nor indeed did any inflammation set in [...] But on the same day in some cases, in others on the following day, and in the rest not many days later, a bubonic swelling developed [...] below the abdomen, but also inside the armpit, and in some cases also beside the ears, and at different points on the thighs. [...] But from there on marked differences [in the symptoms] developed [...]: with some a deep coma, with others a violent delirium [...].
>
> Death came in some cases immediately, in others after many days: and with some the body broke out with black pustules about as large as a lentil, and these did not survive even one day. [...] With many also a vomiting of blood ensued [...] and [...] brought death.[6]

While not all of the symptoms are recognizably those of the Bubonic Plague (which is why the causality has been rejected by some), it should be noted that Procopius, too, wrote in a tradition that was inspired by Thucydides' description of a 'plague' during the Peloponnesian War (431-404 BC). In this narrative a disease spreads from Ethiopia and people are suddenly afflicted. The symptoms are sneezing and hoarseness, as well as chest pains, spasm and memory loss. Thucydides describes how this epidemic leads to the loss of public order, and the lack of care for the sick.[7] Paul Slack emphasises that Thucydides' account introduces some key ideas which become stock ingredients of plague narratives: breakdown of order, turning to or from gods, failure of doctors and the flight of those who fear contagion.[8]

This does not change the fact that the impact of epidemics was real and had wide-ranging consequences for those affected. The impact of the Justinian Plague is said to have resulted in widespread depopulation and changes in the power balance of the eastern Mediterranean - some even associate the rise of Islam to the power vacuum which was created by the fallout of the disease in Byzantium.[9] Disease is surely never the sole reason for change, but it

has on a few occasions been a major contributor to wide-reaching changes. For example, scholars have argued that the Antonine Plague (AD 165–80), which may have been either measles or smallpox, wiped out the population of the Roman Empire to such an extent - up to one half of the people in some areas - that towns and fields stood empty. This epidemic, which continued to flare up for decades, left Rome open to invasion for the next hundred years.[10]

The impact of epidemics in medieval Europe so far has been mainly studied by historians - and the main focus has been the 'Black Death' (1347-53), for which Ole Benedictow's work is still regarded as authoritative.[11] The 14th-century pandemic is a good example of the problems faced by anybody studying medieval disease. Until recently, little was known about the pathogen that caused the disease and scholars have variously 'proved' or 'disproved' that the 14th-century pandemic was caused by plague.[12] Some scholars have claimed that the association of plague with Black Death is misleading, since the epidemic was, according to them, caused by something different.[13] New research shows that there is at least the potential for earlier outbreaks of the plague in Europe. The claim by some historians that the Justinian Plague was indeed a variation of the Black Death may be corroborated by the research of a French team of bioarchaeologists led by Didier Raoult, who reported the successful extraction of ancient mDNA from early medieval plague victims in Germany.[14] However, this evidence has been greeted with scepticism by other epidemiologists, since the results could not be replicated.[15] Genotyping of *Yersinia pestis* DNA has shown that both the Black Death pandemic of the 14th century and the Justinian plague were indeed caused by *Yersinia pestis*.[16]

Arguments about the nature of the diseases in question have mainly focused on the presence or absence of black rats (*Rattus rattus*), thought to be the prime vector of the flea *Xenopsylla cheops,* which is host to the mycobacterium *Yersinia pestis*, and the climate: all plague pandemics have shown seasonal peak periods, even though these may differ between regions. The main problem of defining the type of illness is that the cause of plague, the bacterium *Yersinia pestis,* appears to have mutated over the course of subsequent outbreaks, so that the appearance and severity of the disease varies between them. In recent examinations it has been shown that the medieval plague was indeed caused by a variant strand of *Yersinia pestis* which is now extinct.[17] *Yersinia pestis* itself is a mutation of a (less dangerous) gastro-intestinal bacterium *Yersinia pseudotuberculosis,* which seems to have developed different forms from the earliest known beginnings.[18]

---

[6] Dewing 1914 vol 2, 452-61.
[7] Crawley 1903, 2.47.1-55.1.
[8] Slack 1992, 9.
[9] Little 2007, 16.

[10] Crawford 2007, 78-9.
[11] Benedictow 2004.
[12] Twigg 1984; Benedictow 1992; Scott and Duncan 2004; Sallares 2007; Cohn 2008.
[13] Scott and Duncan 2004, 185-90.
[14] Raoult *et al* 2000; Wiechmann and Gruppe 2005; Drancourt *et al* 2007.
[15] Nutton 2008, 9-10.
[16] Tran *et al* 2011, 493; Hufthammer and Walløe 2013, 1752.
[17] Schuenemann *et al* 2011.
[18] People living in regions in which pigs and rodents have been infected

To add to the complexities, the course of the disease can take different forms: from the relatively 'benign' bubonic plague with a mere 50-60% mortality, to the rarer, but almost 100% lethal, pneumonic plague, depending on whether the lymphatic system or the lungs are infected. Symptoms differ greatly: with bubonic plague, which is caught from flea bites, the infected areas develop painful and dark buboes after three to five days. The bacteria multiply and spread via the lymphatic system. The body's reaction to the infection is high fever and delirium and occasional skin lesions. Pneumonic plague, which is spread by droplet infection, is either caught as a primary infection or as a further complication of bubonic plague, and is characterised by a very short incubation period, high fever and the spewing of blood. The descriptions of symptoms by laymen can therefore resemble anything from tuberculosis to smallpox.

The recent research by Anne Karin Hufthammer and Lars Walløe has shown that rats are no longer the culprit of transmission, and that the disease could be transmitted by humans through lice and fleas carried on the body or in the cloths that they traded.[19] These animals can survive for a long period without feeding and are able to be transported over long distances.[20] Previously it was assumed that only 'blocked' fleas (those who digest the bacterium as a block and regurgitate it into the wound) such as *Xenopsylla cheops*, were carriers, which means that areas without evidence for a large contemporary rodent population (such as Scandinavia) were taken out of the equation.[21] However, recent research has shown that the human flea *Pulex irritans* can also be a transmitter.[22] *Pulex irritans* is ubiquitous and fleas have been found all around the Norse world. They do not need rats as a host, but can be transmitted via dogs, cats and other animals, as well as being harboured in cloth.

There are, to date, no finds of plague DNA from Viking Age skeletons. The main indicators for a spread of the Justinian Plague northwards therefore come from written sources. This is problematic since many of them, such as the *Anglo-Saxon Chronicle* and the *Irish Annals,* are not contemporaneous for the period between AD 570 and 750, when the Justinian Plague supposedly spread across Europe. While the factual accuracy of medieval chronicles is often a point of debate, this adds another layer of complexity, since many descriptions of disease are essentially retrospective and we need to consider how well - and more importantly, to what purpose - these events were remembered.

Historical sources

Medieval Europe saw the emergence of many well-known infectious diseases, such as measles, smallpox and plague, and we may assume that their appearance would not have gone unnoticed. However, records are patchy, and it seems that for many chroniclers there was no compulsion to record *every* outbreak of disease. Instead, there are sporadic accounts - in many cases to make a point, but presumably also when the outbreak was unusual. We are therefore seldom able to chart the path of an epidemic from one place to another.

Not all historical sources are equally interested in outbreaks of disease. Among Frankish sources it is predominantly Gregory of Tours who describes numerous outbreaks of infectious disease in his lifetime (AD 539–94). Gregory tells of a devastating disease which ravaged the Auvergne in 571.[23] The disease was preceded by a comet and he describes how the 'dead were so numerous that one could not count them' and that the church of St Peter in Clermont-Ferrand buried over 300 in one day. The disease, he says, was indicated by a sore under the armpit and in the groin. Another epidemic outbreak manifesting itself in 'boils and tumours' affected Paris in 592,[24] again foreshadowed by 'terrible portents', such as bloody rain. Marseilles, then as now one of the most important sea gateways, was ravaged in 588 and the disease spread as far as Lyon.[25] Gregory states that the infection was first spread through goods purchased from a ship that had come from Spain, and notes that the disease did not spread immediately, but eventually resembled *in segetem flamma accensa,* a 'cornfield set on fire'.[26] It was to return a number of times. Other Frankish sources refer to a 'plague' that affected Spain for seven years during the 7th century (among other calamities) in the *Vita Auduoini,*[27] but there is no description of symptoms, and this may just be a gratuitous mention in a list of (biblical) calamities. Equally unspecific is the disease which is reported in the revised version of the *Royal Frankish Annals,* where an advance against the invading Avars in AD 791 was thwarted because of the pestilence that broke out among the troops and which barely left ten percent alive.[28] The *Annals of St Bertin* tell us that a 'pestilence' carried off a large part of the Frankish population in 856 and struck again in Mainz in 858, which of course, is a period in which Frankish kings also fight off Viking incursions.[29]

Written sources are eclectic - and often disease is only mentioned in the context of other events. For example, one of the most virulent outbreaks of what some scholars regard as plague in England, in 664, is only noteworthy to Bede because it was the cause of the East Saxons lapsing

---

by *Yersinia pseudotuberculosis* are markedly more resistant to the plague (McCormick 2007, 312), and the presence of this in ancient DNA may help answer the question of why some areas seem to have been spared the disease.

[19] Hufthammer and Walløe 2013.
[20] Hufthammer and Walløe 2013, 1758.
[21] Karlsson 1996.
[22] Carniel 2008, 117; Tran *et al* 2011, 493.

[23] *History* iv, 31 - Krusch and Levison 1951, 165
[24] *History* vi.14 - Krusch and Levison 1951, 284.
[25] ix. 21 - Krusch and Levison 1951, 441.
[26] ix. 22 - Krusch 1885, 442.
[27] Fouracre and Gerberding 1996, 158.
[28] Scholz 1970, 70.
[29] Nelson 1991, 81; *ibid* 85.

into paganism.[30] While the nature and spread of it remains unclear, it seems to have had exceptionally high mortality. This disease did not only affect England, but has also been recorded in Irish annals as well (*Annals of Ulster, Annals of Tigernach and Annals of Clonmacnoise*),[31] where it caused *mortalitas magna*, 'great mortality', over the next two years, according to the annalists. The *Annals of the Four Masters* have the following entry:

> A great mortality prevailed in Ireland this year, which was called the *Buidhe Connail*, and the following number of the saints of Ireland died of it: St. Feichin, Abbot of Fobhar, on the 14th of February; St. Ronan, son of Bearach; St. Aileran the Wise; St. Cronan, son of Silne; St. Manchan, of Liath; St. Ultan Mac hUi Cunga, Abbot of Cluain Iraird *Clonard*; Colman Cas, Abbot of Cluain Mic Nois; and Cummine, Abbot of Cluain Mic Nois.[32]

The disease seems to kill indiscriminately, and among its victims are churchmen and kings of Ireland. Adamnan's *Vita Columbani* tells that the community of St Columba in the 670s was spared from *mortalitate, quae nostris temporibus terrarum orbem bis ex parte vastaverat maiore* (a disease which twice in our time devastated large parts of the world). He names the affected areas as 'Italia, the *civitas* of Rome, the transalpine parts of Gaul, Spain, Ireland and Britain, but not Scotland and Pictish regions'.[33] The *Annals of Ulster* tell of a 'great famine' in 670 which followed the epidemic.[34] Whether these two events are related is not specified, but usually there is a shortage of labour to work the land after an epidemic. The consequences of disease are even more pronounced in the *Chronica Scotorum* which reports that the 'great pestilence' of 825, which affected the old and weak, was followed by famine. This is also the year in which much of Ireland was affected by Viking raids.[35] According to this chronicle, as well other texts, this is the beginning of increased Viking activity in Ireland.[36]

In England there are renewed outbreaks of disease well into the 690s. While it is unclear whether they are the same or different diseases, one of the most famous victims is St Æþelðryð, who according to Bede died of plague in 680.[37] Welsh annals, such as the *Chronicle of Princes* (*Brut y Tywysogion*) report outbreaks of disease in Ireland for 684,[38] and the *Annales Cambriae* report that a great plague was suffered in Britain in 682 and Ireland in 683.[39] It seems that the 7th century was a time of repeated outbreaks of disease, which in Ireland seemed to have recurred until well into the 8th century, since the *Annals*

of Ulster in particular tell of several diseases that affected the country.[40] It is, however, apparent that these are not one, but several different afflictions, ranging from *pestis qui dicitur Baccach cum uentris profluuio* (a plague named *Bacchach* with dysentery) in the *Annals of Ulster* for 709, to *bolgach* which is 'rampant' in 743.[41] The nature of these diseases remains subject to debate, since the names of the diseases seem to primarily refer to colours.[42]

The 9th century sees at least three serious outbreaks of disease: in Ireland in 806, when according to the *Annals of Ulster* 'great pestilence' breaks out, and again in 825, when *magna pestilentia* is followed by famine;[43] in England *ceapes cwilde & monna* (disease of cattle and people)[44] in 897, which according to the *Anglo-Saxon Chronicle* killed many of King Alfred's thegns.[45] Would such sickness have had any impact on the king's campaigning?

The 10th century sees further outbreaks of disease in Britain and Ireland, some of which seem to affect large areas. For example, in 987 the *Annals of Ulster* record that 'St Vitus' Dance' affected all of Britain, Ireland and 'Saxonland'.[46] The Vikings in Dublin, according to the *Annals of the Four Masters*, suffered an outbreak of 'bloody flux' in 949.[47] A new disease, evocatively called *scitta*, which kills many, is recorded in English sources for the year 987 by Simeon of Durham.[48] The name suggests an outbreak of dysentery. Interestingly, while Ireland sees several outbreaks of disease, cattle murrain and famine in the mid-10th century, this does not seem to affect Anglo-Saxon England, which is unusual. The period of stability under Kings Æthelstan and Edgar seems to be mirrored in a healthy population, and surely such varied reporting shows that disease is part of a larger picture painted by the chroniclers.

The language of disease

It is apparent from the list above that the chroniclers knew about different diseases. It is not always clear if these refer to any recognizable condition. Generally, palaeopathologists are wary of posthumous diagnoses made from written sources. Too often, these sources are not descriptive, but steeped in the ideology of their time, which means that the vocabulary and images used by the writers may be based on what contemporary writers regarded as authoritative. Disease in many of these accounts has a didactic function, as for example, a passage from Adamnan's 8th-century *Vita Columbani,* in which the saint, exiled on Iona, sends aid to his fellow Irish, who are subjected to a pestiferous cloud affecting humans and cattle.[49] Healing occurs with

[30] Colgrave and Mynors 1969 3.27,310.
[31] Mac Airt and Mac Niocaill 1983, 134-7.
[32] Ryan and O'Donovan 2002, 277.
[33] Fowler 1894, 125.
[34] Mac Airt and Mac Niocaill 1983, 139.
[35] Hennessey and Mac Niocaill 2010, 109.
[36] See also Ó Corráin 1998.
[37] Colgrave and Mynors 1969 4.19, 392.
[38] Jones 1955, 2.
[39] *Annales Cambriae* in Morris 1980, 46.

[40] For a list see Bonser 1963, 61.
[41] Mac Airt and Mac Niocaill 1983, 166; *ibid,* 198.
[42] Bonser 1963, 64-72.
[43] Mac Airt and Mac Niocaill 1983, 260; *ibid,* 282.
[44] Dumville and Keynes 1983: variant spelling in MS BCD is *cwyld.*
[45] Bately 1986, 56.
[46] Mac Airt and Mac Niocaill 1983, 420.
[47] Ryan and O'Donovan 2002, 655.
[48] *Simeon of Durham* in Stephenson 1853, 510.
[49] Fowler 1894, 73-4.

'blessed bread' which shows that this episode is supposed to underline the saint's powers to perform miracles, rather than to present an account of actual disease. Conversely, the fact that chroniclers wrote in the conventions of their time may present us with evidence, if we learn the language that chroniclers apply to describe epidemics. Pestiferous clouds, comets and other natural phenomena are often connected with outbreaks of disease in historical sources, to the point that comets may be gratuitously added to some Anglo-Saxon texts in order to indicate calamity.[50] Few people who have commented on the famous 'dragons in the sky' episode of 793 in the *Anglo-Saxon Chronicle* have noted that this passage is also a precursor for a period of great hunger, not just Vikings.[51]

The association of comets with calamity goes as far back as Isidore, who writes in the *Etymologies*: 'A comet is a star, so named because it spreads out the hair of its light. When this type of star appears it signifies plague, famine, or war'.[52] It is possible that the mention of natural phenomena may be linked to outbreaks of disease. David Wood has made a very good case for the Irish annals, where an early copyist of the *Iona Chronicle* misread *glandula* (referring to swelling of glands with bubonic plague) for a diminutive of *glans* - 'acorn'. Subsequent copyists continued to use term 'glut of acorns' when referring to plague outbreaks.[53]

Old English uses a variety of terms for epidemics, including *cwealm*, cognate with *cwelan* 'to die', *cwyld*, as well as *wol*. According to the *Dictionary of Old English*,[54] *cwealm* has a number of meanings, and only one of them is 'pestilence'. In texts it can be part of a stock phrase *hungor and cwealm* describing divine judgement. This is used particularly in homiletic and religious writings,[55] such as Ælfric's homily for the second Sunday in Advent, in a passage based on Gregory the Great's depiction of celestial signs as a token of impending *pestilentia*: '*Mid cwealme and mid hunger we sind gelome geswencte*' (With disease and with hunger we are frequently chastised).[56] In other instances, *cwealm* refers to specific outbreaks in the past. The majority of texts in which *cwealm* appears are homilies, but the term is also applied to outbreaks of disease in the year 664 in the E-Version of the *Anglo-Saxon Chronicle*.[57]

The compound *manncwealm* (epidemic) is used as an alternative in the 664 entry of the *Chronicle* and appears in the A, C, D and F versions. Generally *man(n)cwealm* is used - other than in the *Chronicle* versions - to refer to

diseases sent by God to test humans, as for example, in Wærferth's translation of Gregory the Great's *Dialogues*.[58] *Cwyld* glosses Latin *pestis* in a number of instances, such as the Old English version of the *Rule of St Chrodegang*, in a passage which states that an 'improper' priest ought to be abhorred *swilce uncoðu oððe cwyld* (like disease and plague) which is an extension of the Latin which simply states *pestis*. *Cwyld* also glosses the Latin cognate *lue*, as for example in the Old English gloss to Sedulius' *Carmen Paschale*.[59] Its compounds *cwyldbære* (pestiferous) and *cwyldeflod* (death-bringing flood), which refers to Noah's flood, underline the impression that *cwyld* is not just devastating, but also wide-ranging.

Other terms seem to be text-generic. *Wol* or *wool* are especially used in translations of Bede's *Ecclesiastical History*, as well as in the Old English *Orosius*, where they refer to epidemics in history. The term can refer to epidemics that affect both humans and animals, and glosses Latin *pestilentia* and *lues* in the Old English glosses to Aldhelm's *De laude virginitatis*.[60] What many of these terms have in common is that they do not refer to actual outbreaks of disease but describe events that have significant moral overtones.

Old Irish historical sources have a number of terms for the various epidemics that affected early medieval Ireland, many of them obscure. Among the terms are *buidhe co[n] nail*, reported for the year 664 in the *Annals of the Four Masters*,[61] which is given as *mortalitas* in the *Annals of Ulster*.[62] The term *buide* can mean yellow in Irish,[63] and on this basis several scholars have argued that this is some form of jaundice or 'yellow pestilence'.[64] There is another 'yellow' disease: *cron chonaill* (saffron disease) in the year 555 of the *Annals of Ulster*, where it is cited alongside *Buidhe Chonaill*.[65] Other infectious diseases are named *blefed*, *bolgach* and *samthrosc*. These have been identified as smallpox (*bolgach*, for example 577 in the *Annals of Innisfallen*),[66] or plague (*blefed*).[67] It is extremely difficult to determine the nature of these diseases from the limited information given in the texts. Anne Dooley has recently offered an etymological reading, which moves away from interpreting the yellow colour associated with a number of these terms as a token of the symptoms to a more generic explanation that shows the colour refers to ill-health and is thus a generic term for epidemics.[68] Other diseases, such as *baccach*, which translates as 'lame' in the *Annals of Ulster* entry for 708,[69] have been interpreted as poliomyelitis,[70]

[50] Keynes 1992, 161.
[51] (ms FDE).
[52] *Cometes stella dicta est, eo quod comas luminis fundat ex se. Quod genus sideris quando apparuerit, aut pestilentiam, aut famem, aut bella significat* (Barney *et al* 2006, 105).
[53] Wood 2004, 499.
[54] *Dictionary of Old English A - G online*: diPaolo Healey *et al.* 2007, http://tapor.library.utoronto.ca/doe/ [accessed 26/4/2010]; abbreviated *DOE* from here on with date of access).
[55] *DOE* 27/4/2010.
[56] Clemoes 1997, 525. The verb *swincan* means 'toil', but I think that *swingan* 'to chastise' fits the sense better.
[57] Irvine 2004, 30.

[58] Hecht 1900, 192.
[59] Merritt 1945.
[60] The data are taken from the di Paolo 2009 - *Old English Corpus*: http://tapor.library.utoronto.ca/doecorpus/ [accessed 8/3/2013].
[61] Ryan and O'Donovan 2002, 276.
[62] *ibid* 134.
[63] Toner 2007 - eDIL: accessed 10/6/2010.
[64] Bonser 1963, 67.
[65] Ryan and O'Donovan 2002, 78.
[66] Mac Airt and Färber 2008, 77.
[67] cf Bonser 1963, 81.
[68] Dooley 2007, 218.
[69] Ryan and O'Donovan 2002, 166.
[70] Bonser 1963, 83.

but it is linked in the annal to *uentris profluuio* ((out) flowing of the stomach), which is most likely dysentery, and therefore a different disease.

Early medieval historical records thus present us with a variety of diseases, which may or may not be variants of some of the most lethal infectious diseases. It is interesting that later medieval texts which are written or compiled around the time of the Black Death are often no more precise in the linguistic terminology. The medieval Icelandic annals, albeit making use of some English sources, such as Bede's *Historia Ecclesiastica,* are not primarily interested in epidemics outside Iceland. However, since much of the early material is copied from Latin sources, they retain some information, such as the arrival of a comet and an outbreak of *manndávr mikill* (great mortality) for the year 542,[71] as well as an epidemic in Byzantium in 531: *mandauðr a þesso are.*[72] The annals are the product of the High and Late Middle Ages and during this period they do provide contemporary information on disease such as the 14th-century *Lögmanns Annáll:*

> *J þenna tima kom drep sott so mickil vm alla nordr halfu heimsins at alldre kom slik fyrr sidan londin bygduzst. fyrst kom sottin vpp i Babilone [...]. þatt var kyn sottarinnar at menn lifdu eige meirr en eitt dægr edr tuo. med hordum stinga. after þat sætte at blod spyiu...*

(At this time came a disease to all of the northern hemisphere which was so great that none such had come before nor since to the inhabited world. The disease first arrived in Babylon [...]. That was the kind of disease where people lived no more than a day or two with sincere [stabbing] pains, and after that spew blood.)[73]

Just as in most Old Norse sources, and especially in the Icelandic Annals, the diseases are called by the generic term *sótt* (disease). This word is generally used for all kinds of infectious disease, sometimes prefixed by the particular part of the anatomy which is most affected, as, for example, *kverka sótt* (throat disease) in the 1310 entry of *Skálholts Annaler.*[74] Unlike other medieval texts, the annals do not moralize disease. Outbreaks are not punishments for transgressions or tests of faith, but are, like famine and other disasters, noted by the annalists (who often give information on outbreaks in other places as well). Additionally, the term *drepsótt* 'mortality' (literally, killing disease) is used to denote epidemics, and occasionally the annalist talks of *manndauðr* (mortality), as for example in the entry in the *Annales vetustissimi* for 1310:

> *Drepsott ok manndauðr um alltan vestfirðinga fiorðung ok sunnlendinga fiorðung ok bólna sott sva at sumir menn fvnoðo i svndr*

(Epidemic and mortality in all of the West Fjords quarter and in the South quarter, and *bólna sott*, so bad that some people rotted apart [away?].)[75]

The term *bólna sótt* is commonly translated as 'smallpox' by analogy with modern Icelandic *bólusótt* (variola, smallpox). However, the word *bola* in Old Icelandic, on which the term is based, can indicate a 'blister' or even the boss of a shield. It is etymologically related to Modern German *Beule* and English 'boil'. The textual evidence here seems to suggest that the flesh of these people rotted away, and perhaps we should consider that this disease may be different from the modern versions of smallpox, or may indeed have been used for any disease that left the afflicted with visible skin lesions, including bubonic plague.

The Icelandic annals do not just note outbreaks of disease, but like other chronicles, on occasion they tell us about the mortality of the disease. For example, an outbreak of *bólna sótt* in 1347 is described like this in the *Annals of Skálholt:*

> *Bolna sótt hin fiorða um allt land, sva mikil at engi var sva gamall at slika myndi [...] Gekk sóttin fyrir sunnan land þetta arit enn it siðarra fyrir norðan; for hon sva gersamliga yfir sveitirnar at hon tok naliga hvern yngra mann enn fertugan, ok marga ellri. ok iafnvel var bolan a bórnunum þeim er moðirin fæddi viðr andlát sítt.*

(The fourth *bólna sótt* in all of the country, so big that no-one so old that they could remember such like [...] The disease struck in the south of the country this year but in the next it went north. It spread so thoroughly through districts that it took nearly every person younger than forty and many older [ones]. And there were 'boils' as well on the children who were delivered when their mother gave birth at her death.)[76]

Whether the pathogen of *bólna sótt* is variola or not, the fact that this disease decimates much of Iceland the year before the outbreak of the plague in Europe, may be significant. *Lögmanns Annáll* adds that 'this disease' - referring to the plague - did not come to Iceland in this year: *þessi sott kom ecki aa Island,*[77] but it does not mean that the island was spared. In the 14th century Iceland was ruled from Norway, and trade and travel with the island was strictly regulated. Such sanctions may have given Iceland a respite. As seen with some of the Frankish outbreaks, trade ships did not just bring goods, but often harboured much deadlier cargo. The annals record that in 1379 a ship came to Iceland and

---

[71] *Annales regii*, Storm 1888, 91.
[72] *Annales Reseniani*, Storm 1888, 9.
[73] *Lögmanns annáll*, Storm 1888, 275.
[74] Storm 1888, 203.

[75] Storm 1888, 53.
[76] Storm 1888, 213.
[77] Storm 1888, 276.

that *bolna sott* affected the whole country which resulted in *mikill manndaudr* (great mortality).[78] Equally, it is possible that the fact that *bólna sótt* had already decimated a good proportion of the vulnerable population may have prevented the plague from finding many victims.

The Old Norse term *plága,* derived from classical Latin *plaga* (stroke), initially denoted a wound,[79] but acquired the meaning 'plague, nuisance', as evident in the 1402 entries in two of the Icelandic annals, possibly by analogy with biblical 'plagues': in modern Icelandic this is the standard term for the plague. The word 'plague' for biblical calamities had been established in other languages as well, such as Wycliffe's 1382 Bible translation. Some scholars have argued that plague did not arrive in Iceland before the early 15th century,[80] when, for example, the annalists in the *Oddveria Annall* and *Gottskalks Annall* mention the word *plaga* in the 1402 entry. Other annals, however, continue to use established terminology, such as *manndáuðr*.[81] It appears that tradition, rather than medical accuracy, guides the annalist here. The depictions of later epidemics show that authors work in a tradition of writing about disease. While the Icelandic annalist does not use 'plague' to moralize, some of descriptions continue to use established images. While medically the 14th century plague, the Justinian Plague and any of the medieval 'plagues' may be different, we may be able to use the imagery and vocabulary to show similarities and differences.

A question of numbers

In order to establish if any of the above named diseases could have led to a wide-spread depopulation which allowed for renewed settlement, we need to know just how many people lived and died during this period. However, one of the most difficult questions to answer for this period is the case fatality rates of diseases. Generally, modern scientists differentiate between virgin (first) outbreaks of infectious disease which are usually very virulent, and later outbreaks, which affect fewer people since some part of the population has already developed immunity. Unless there is a mutation in the pathogen, survivors of a disease will be immune to recurrent outbreaks and thus the epidemic will eventually run out of 'fuel'. Since there are no reliable demographic documents, we may approach the question of the number of dead in the outbreaks of the 7th and 8th centuries by looking at contemporaneous data from other areas. It has been assumed that population in Frankia nearly trebled between the 6th and the 7th century,[82] which has been calculated on the number of dead bodies in cemeteries from the period. Helena Hamerow observes that the increase in the number of dead is too steep for a natural population growth and concludes that the reason behind this rise is that the people brought under

Frankish overlordship adopted a more readily datable model of burial.[83] However, could it be that the increase in the numbers of dead may also be the result of more people dying contemporaneously?

The problem with establishing a case for or against outbreaks of epidemics is that diseases very rarely occur in a vacuum, and that in a largely agrarian society the fallout from them may be even deadlier than the initial pandemic. 'Plague' is never just the disease alone, it is abetted by climatic changes (which means that immunity was already low because of bad harvests) and succeeded by economic problems (a shortage of labour means that fields are not ploughed, so famine is a consequence). For example, the *Annals of Ulster* tell of a cattle murrain in 778 which leads to a 'mortality of people from want', and is followed by an outbreak of *bolggach* 'smallpox'.[84] It is interesting that Harris Lines (which can include malnutrition) are observed more frequently in bodies from the Middle Anglo-Saxon period,[85] which is the period for which chronicles and annals tell of repeated outbreaks of disease.

Many medieval societies, however, were conservative in the ways they used the land and in some cases, such as in areas of predominant animal husbandry, there may not be any easily detectable changes. A case study from medieval Iceland has shown that the medieval population of Skarftártunga, southern Iceland, hit doubly by the plague and rapid climate change, continued to farm in their usual way.[86] The authors of this study conclude that since livestock is not immediately impacted by human disease, they continue to graze the land in the usual way.

Disease does not strike indiscriminately, however: unlike 'normal' mortality patterns, where death rates are highest in early childhood and old age, population statistics from pandemics show significant death levels among adolescent and mature people. However, infectious diseases only kill once, so that those who have survived the disease will have immunity and any renewed outbreak will predominantly affect children and the young. Thus populations may not recover for a long time. The 8th and 9th centuries in Anglo-Saxon England saw large changes, not just in burial archaeology, but also in the restructuring of agriculture and the establishment of central places. Excavation has shown that some villages, such as Mucking (Essex) and West Heslerton (Yorkshire), were abandoned, but often only to be replaced by new villages just a few miles down the road. The old explanation that Anglo-Saxon England was greatly disrupted by 'Viking' activity is an overstatement. Many of the fundamental changes that took place in the Middle Anglo-Saxon period are part of new power structures, where religious and secular authority converged in the hands of fewer, but more influential, rulers. The incoming Scandinavians, as Dawn Hadley and others have shown,[87]

---

[78] *Lögmanns annáll,* Storm 1888, 281; *Flatey annáll,* Storm 1888, 413.
[79] Buntrock 2003, 67.
[80] Benedictow 2004; Karlsson 1996.
[81] *Lögmanns Annáll,* Storm 1888, 287.
[82] Hamerow 2002, 107.

[83] Hamerow 2002, 108.
[84] Mac Airt and Mac Niocaill 1983, 232.
[85] Cox and Roberts 2003, 188.
[86] Streeter *et al* 2012, 3666.
[87] Hadley 2007.

were more likely to 'fit in' than to disrupt. There has been a longstanding debate about the number of settlers that came during the 9th century, but the wealth of place-name evidence suggests that there were speaker communities that lasted long enough to name or rename many places with Scandinavian elements, and we should suggest that the settlement included a substantial body of people. The easy transition into English life also suggests that in many cases the incomers were not as unwelcome as suggested by written sources, such as the *Anglo-Saxon Chronicle*. Could these incomers have replenished a population which had been disrupted or held back by repeated waves of disease?

Bones and bodies

If there have been epidemics, where are the bodies? Where are the plague pits and the mass graves? The question of numbers is especially problematic, since only a fraction of the overall dead can ever be recovered from any historical period.[88] Bodies decay and not everybody gets buried in the first place: some may be cremated, others left to decay - particularly in rural settings where there is no immediate danger of contaminating the neighbours. In evaluations of epidemics, we should consider that infectious diseases kill too quickly to leave signatures on the bone. The presence of disease can in many cases only be shown with costly ancient DNA analysis, if at all, since even other indicators of disease, such as stress patterns on the long bones (Harris Lines) may be caused by other factors, such as malnutrition.[89] Finding the dead is made more difficult since attempts to prevent contagion may have led to a quick disposal of the body, which for this reason may not be included in the usual burial ground. The necessity to find quick burial solutions is evidenced in later medieval sources, such as the Icelandic annals, which tell us that so many people died during the Black Death in France that graves could not be dug for them. Pope Clement VI therefore consecrated the river Rhone so that they could be disposed of in it.[90] For a long time it has been difficult to locate the bodies of plague victims even in the relatively well documented 14th century, and this is even more complex for potential earlier populations. While a large fraction of Anglo-Saxon cemeteries contained multiple inhumations, there are very rarely more than three bodies buried in the same grave, and in many cases their inhumation was not simultaneous. A rare burial of five people at Bifrons, Kent is too early to be considered as representing victims of this plague, but the inhumation of five people in one grave at Sedgeford, Norfolk may fit. Andrew Reynolds has suggested that the Viking Age charnel grave at Repton, which contains over 264 individuals showing little evidence of trauma, may have been from a plague pit.[91]

At Edix Hill, Cambridgeshire, a group of bodies dated to the 6th century were buried in a ditch, one of which, G

66, shows signs of having suffered from tuberculosis.[92] While this person clearly is a 'survivor' - i.e. the initial infection did not kill them - it points to the possibility that the infected were given different forms of burial. Such a distinction has been suggested for the 'missing' plague pits of the Black Death: 'The archaeological evidence for plague is remarkable scanty, considering its recurrence over the centuries'.[93] Plague pits from Black Death outbreaks are remarkably hard to locate, despite the fact that they are copiously described in written sources and depicted in images of the time. The expansion of major European cities in recent centuries has not led to a discovery of mass burials which could be associated with epidemics, and it has been suggested that many corpses may have been cremated.[94] Roberta Gilchrist has suggested that ash or charcoal deposits around dead bodies may stem from a fear of the contagious corpses of plague victims walking and this folkloristic element survives well into the 14th century, when many plague graves at the London cemetery of East Smithfields show hearth ash being included.[95] Cremation burial was abandoned during the Middle Anglo-Saxon period, which saw a strong theological and legal focus on the body, dead or alive. Cremation makes good sense in terms of prevention of further disease, and ash or charcoal deposits may signify that the mourners wished to utilize the protective aspects of fire while adhering to the standard burial rite of their time. Victoria Thompson, who examined charcoal burial in later Anglo-Saxon England, connects the rite with penance, which is not necessarily contradictory.[96] She states that charcoal burial, which she dates from the 9th century onwards, is more common at larger minsters and that it can vary in prevalence at a single site.[97]

Generally, epidemics require a large group of people to 'thrive', otherwise the disease will quickly run its course for a lack of new victims.[98] However, this means that when the disease returns there is no or little immunity in the population and mortality rates remain high, unlike pandemics which can 'feed' on large groups of people where the survivors had longer exposure to the pathogens.[99] Therefore every subsequent outbreak is almost as virulent as the first. Repeat outbreaks will have some impact on populations, since every wave will result in a small, but significant dip. Such variations are of course, much harder to find and at a time when famine and war almost regularly decimated populations we need to find better ways of identifying the plague dead.

In this light, should we actually expect mass graves, or should we rather look for a series of unusual burials over time? The *Annals of Fulda* are rare in describing the burial

[88] Waldron 2007.
[89] Signoli 2012, 221.
[90] Storm 1888, 223 [*Skálholt*]; 275 [*Lögmanns*]; 404 [*Flatøy*].
[91] Reynolds 2009.
[92] Duhig 1998, 184.
[93] Nutton 2008, 9.
[94] Nutton 2008, 9.
[95] Gilchrist 2008, 145, 150-1.
[96] Thompson 2004, 117-22.
[97] *ibid*, 119-20.
[98] Benedictow 1996, 173.
[99] Cliff *et al* 2007.

of the victims, pointing out that an outbreak of disease in Bavaria of 883 was so severe that 'often two bodies were buried in one grave', which suggests that this was a rather unusual event.[100] Annia Cherryson has recently observed that some burial grounds of south-west England had a tendency to densely pack burials from the Middle Anglo-Saxon period onwards.[101] Graves were re-opened and bodies were tightly squeezed into place. She associates this with changes in Church regulations, which enclosed churchyards and left little room for later burial.[102] However, could these practices also signify a need for rapid burial in an established place? There is an interesting question of who is to be included in such prestigious ground and who should be excluded. Increasingly, 'sinners' are excluded from consecrated ground, which suggests that those who died without penance may not be included.[103] However, Anglo-Saxon homilists are careful in their evaluation of disease, which in some examples signifies being favoured by God. Epidemics are sent to 'test' people, but this does not turn their victims automatically into villains. In terms of disease prevention, quick and unceremonious burial may be necessary and we may consider whether some burials which have been labelled as 'deviant', such as prone burials in the Middle Anglo-Saxon period, were actually the result of a hasty burial of the body wrapped in a shroud, with the result that the position of the corpse is more or less accidental.

However, if we expect that there is an alternative burial for the afflicted, where would we find the 'unusual' dead? There is a small, but significant number of burials associated with Middle to late Anglo-Saxon settlements.[104] These are often 'deviant' burials, and while not all of them may be those of people who succumbed to disease, it could be possible that these are people who died suddenly and where a quick disposal of the body was essential. The fact that they were buried away from hallowed ground, but not with execution burials, could indicate that these people died without receiving the essential deathbed rituals, such as confession.

In any case, epidemics must have led to some disruptions of communities. John Maddicot claims that we may measure the impact of the northern arm of the Justinian Plague by looking at its effects on settlements such as Mucking and West Stow. His idea, first published in 1997, that pandemics fundamentally changed the face of Anglo-Saxon England has never been followed up. The dating of his archaeological evidence is complex; for example, it is clear that the cemetery at Mucking was given up in the 7th century, but the settlement continued into the 8th century. It is assumed that the population was now buried at the nearby St Cedd in Tilbury.[105] In a few places we observe that settlements are given up but new places appear only a

few kilometres away, as for example West Heslerton, which was abandoned in the 9th century, but could have been replaced by nearby Wharram Percy (Yorkshire). Middle Anglo-Saxon England also sees increasing urbanization, which implies a growing population in at least in some areas.

This rise in numbers may confirm Maddicot's claims that populations recovered quickly after the plague outbreak,[106] which is contradictory to observations from 14th-century outbreaks of plague, where populations did not recover until well into the 16th century and in some areas of Scandinavia not even until the 18th century. The medieval plague outbreaks in Iceland had devastating effects, even for those who survived the disease. Gunnar Karlsson shows that even though a reduced workforce may have hung on to farms, 40 years after the first outbreak a considerable number of farms were deserted, in some parts more than 50%.[107] 15th-century Iceland, unlike 9th-century England, was not subject to migration and even an increased birth rate would not replenish figures. This is different from Anglo-Saxon England, which absorbed waves of Scandinavian migration in the 9th century. The question is whether it is possible to see changes in settlement as a result of an influx of Scandinavians.

Anglo-Saxon settlement archaeology has been relatively neglected in comparison with burial archaeology, and the balance is only just being redressed. A number of important publications, including the settlement at Yarnton (Oxfordshire) and Bloodmore Hill (Suffolk),[108] have greatly advanced our understanding of rural settlements. Many of the excavated Middle and Late Anglo-Saxon settlements had at least one or two bodies associated with them. Often these are buried in pits or boundary ditches. It is debatable why these people were not buried in churchyards or grave fields, and a body underneath the floor boards may suggest a victim of crime, rather than a special deposit. Still there is a remarkable tendency to bury people in ditches, which, even if conducted in the blackest night, could not have gone unnoticed. Examples, such as the 8th-century inhumation of a woman at Higham Ferrers (Northamptonshire),[109] who had, according to the osteologist, been hanged until rotten and partly eaten by dogs,[110] suggest that these may be people who had been deliberately excluded. Location clearly mattered, and it is possible that diseased bodies were also regarded as 'deviant', so that some of the burials in ditches and on boundaries may be those of people who had suffered from infectious disease.

We can observe a number of changes - often quite radical - which affect settlements. Higham Ferrers, for example, was dismantled and cleared some time in the late 8th or early 9th century, which interestingly is approximately

[100] Reuter 1992, 106.
[101] Cherryson 2007.
[102] Cherryson 2007, 137.
[103] Thompson 2004, 171-79.
[104] Hamerow 2006.
[105] Hirst and Clark, 2009.

[106] Maddicot 2007, 214.
[107] Karlsson 1996, 263.
[108] Hey *et al* 2004; Lucy *et al* 2009.
[109] Hardy *et al* 2007.
[110] Witkin in Hardy 2007, 141-3.

the period in which the human remains were deposited in the ditch.[111] The site was not completely abandoned: some scattered activity is evident after a hiatus, but it never regained the status of a secular centre of power. While Higham Ferrers may have been victim of changing power structures in Middle Anglo-Saxon Northamptonshire, there may also be other reasons that accelerated its demise.

The most significant events of the 9th century in England were undoubtedly the arrival of Viking settlers and the rise to supremacy of Wessex. Traditional history sees Viking migration as a series of 'take-overs', without being able to explain what happened to the indigenous population. This picture has become much more refined of late. James Barrett has recently taken issue with the idea of a Viking 'advance' and favours a 'leapfrog' theory, which proposes that settlement came via previously-established communities of other Scandinavians.[112] The migration of Scandinavians to the British Isles is not exclusive to the Viking Age, and these communities may have used routes that were established well before the Viking Age. For example, stable isotope analyses from the 5th - 7th century burial ground of the North Yorkshire village of West Heslerton indicates that some Scandinavian migrants settled with the Anglo-Saxon population.[113] Future research from stable isotopes may show whether this is an isolated case, or whether pockets of Scandinavian settlers existed alongside their Anglo-Saxon and British neighbours centuries before the beginning of the Viking Age. However, in many cases Viking settlement seems to be away from established Anglo-Saxon settlements. The Norfolk town of Norwich, for example, has only very little evidence for an Early Anglo-Saxon settlement,[114] but sees impressive growth after the arrival of a Viking, or hybrid Anglo-Scandinavian population. Researchers at Norwich were in a position to extract ancient DNA from teeth which were found at the late Saxon cemeteries around Castle Mall.[115] Interestingly, 60% of the haplotypes do not correspond with modern English examples (indicating genetic discontinuity), and at least four different individuals had haplotypes which correspond with those found in Orkney, Iceland and Norway.[116]

The idea that a lack of land forced Viking migration is untenable, even though the Viking Age sees a healthy increase of population,[117] but there are dramatic changes which see the rise of larger towns within the agrarian economies of the north. The sheer volume of archaeological and toponymic evidence from the British Isles shows that they had a place to go. If recurrent waves of epidemic disease in the 7th and 8th centuries had decimated the population so that there were areas left untended, the British Isles would be an attractive destination indeed. Even if there had been no widespread reduction of people, epidemics may have led to a stagnation of existing numbers.

Disease and the end of all things

Migration can be an important factor in sustaining communities, since there is the potential that a population will disappear completely if there is no renewed influx. While a decline in population may have made migration to the British Isles an attractive possibility, the impact of disease is even more evident in the more sparsely populated areas of the Viking diaspora, such as Greenland, where the Norse disappeared after facing the effects of both climate change and disease. The most popular theory for the demise of the Norse population is still Jared Diamond's idea that the Greenland Norse were unable to adapt to their changing environment.[118] More nuanced research, such as that of Andrew Dugmore, has shown that it was not an inability to adapt to the changing climate, but the fallout from a combination of disasters: the Black Death in Norway and Europe, changes in the economy and trade, together with a change in climate, which caused the collapse of the colonies in Greenland.[119]

Studies by Eva Panagiotakopulu and her team on the insect remains from the last days of the Western Settlement in Greenland show that the inhabitants died a slow death from protein poisoning.[120] Isolated by increasingly harsh winters, the diet of the population had essentially been based on hunted animal, especially caribou. A diet based mainly on protein from lean meat means that the body will attack its own fat reserves and it literally 'eat' itself. Research from the farm building shows that after the inhabitants died their remains seems to have been devoured by carrion-eating animals, but that their domestic animals grazed at the farm long after the humans had gone.[121]

The results of excavations from the Norse farmstead at Nipaatsoq are congruent with observations by the priest Ivarr Barðarsson who wrote a report about his visit to Greenland around 1368.[122] His account describes that neither Christian nor heathen were alive at the Western settlement, but he saw domestic animals roaming around. It is clear that the place had been abandoned by the Norse, but was not taken over by the Inuit.

Interestingly, the insect remains from the farm at Nipaasoq, especially around the fireplace, contained high numbers of *Pulex irritans*. The presence of this parasite, which, as stated before, is a known transmitter of plague, does not have to mean that the Western Settlement succumbed to disease, but there is a good chance that the demise of the

[111] Hardy *et al* 2007, 192.
[112] Barrett 2008, 675.
[113] Montgomery *et al* 2005, 134.
[114] Shepherd-Popescu 2009/I, 49. Although a potential 7th- or 8th-century cemetery with an estimated burial population of 43, of which almost half were children (including one infant with Paget's Disease), may have been disturbed by the building of the bailey (Shepherd-Popescu 2009, 255).
[115] Töpf 2009, 253.
[116] Töpf 2009, 253.
[117] Benedictow 1996, 180-81.
[118] Diamond 2006.
[119] Dugmore *et al* 2007.
[120] Panagiotakopulu *et al* 2007, 300-306.
[121] Panagiotakopulu *et al* 2007, 300-306.
[122] Mathers 2009, 81.

Greenland Norse may have been assisted by an outbreak of disease. Perhaps future research should consider whether disease might have potentially have had a hand in the demise of the colony. Ole Benedictow categorically states that there is no proof that the plague ever reached Greenland.[123] I would argue that the plague did not have to reach Greenland to have had a devastating effect, which has also been considered by Lynnerup and others.[124] The effect of the plague on medieval economies, such as the loss of almost 50% of the population in some areas of rural Norway, meant that there was no longer a need to trade with countries that were hazardous to reach. The example from Norse Greenland shows that isolated and sparsely populated communities are vulnerable to outbreaks of disease even though not one member within the community may be directly afflicted.

Conclusion

Currently, the idea that pandemics may have affected northern Europe in the early Middle Ages, and accelerated major changes in population and power structures, is at best hypothetical. In this paper I have presented the evidence that plague may have led to destabilization, if not depopulation of areas that were subsequently settled by Scandinavian incomers. It should be stressed that most changes never just have one cause, and it would be wrong to claim that the Viking Age began because of disease. The examples from medieval chronicles underline that epidemics reduced populations many times prior to the Black Death, and potentially had economic as well as political impact, as well as being a source of anxiety to medieval people. While not all pathogens that caused these epidemics have yet been fully detected, there is good evidence that at least some epidemics were indeed caused by *Yersinia pestis*. We can also note that the authors who described diseases did this in a literary tradition and that this tradition needs to be studied. The vulnerability of small and isolated communities, such as the North Atlantic colonies, made them more prone to disease. Epidemics did not necessarily have to be a primary factor of population decline, as shown in the examples from the Greenlandic medieval settlements, since interruptions of trade coupled with other changes may be enough to extinguish a whole group of people forever. A study of the impact of epidemic in the early medieval samples may draw on the later evidence to show that decline is not always caused by direct infection.

The examination of written texts also shows the limitations of our understanding of disease and the ways in which contemporaries wrote about it. It is time to learn the medieval 'language' of disease, which for many was as terrifying and incomprehensible as many other natural phenomena, and was consequently associated with the supernatural. Other aspects, such as the changes in burial rituals, such as masses for the dead, may also be rooted in the need to treat the dead body differently: to allow memory away from the corpse. We should consider that disease and its fallouts were not only more immediate for medieval populations, but that they were also more ubiquitous. For societies in which good health may have been a bonus rather than the norm, disease was a steady companion, a source of constant sorrow and a force to be reckoned with.

Acknowledgments

Like many Arts-based papers, this essay has had a lengthy genesis and I am fully aware that scientific research is publishing at a rapid pace. I have tried to integrate as much of the latest developments on plague research as possible, but if there is one reason for greater interdisciplinarity, it is the ways in which arts and science can inform each other. I would like to express my sincere thanks to Judith Jesch and Chris Callow who gave me valuable advice on an early draft of this paper and to the anonymous readers for their very helpful comments and suggestions. I would like to thank the CELT team for allowing me to quote from their resource. I would also like to thank Debby Banham for much helpful support during the writing of this paper. All mistakes are mine.

---

[123] Benedictow 2004, 146.
[124] Lynnerup 2003, 142.

Bibliography

Arevalo, F. (ed.) 1850. *De Natura Rerum, Etymologiae*, in *Sancti Isidori, Hispalensis episcopi, Opera omnia*, vol 3. Paris.

Antoine, D. 2008. 'The Archaeology of Plague', in V. Nutton (ed.), *Pestilential Complexities*, 101-14. London: Wellcome Trust Centre for the History of Medicine at UCL.

Barney, S., Lewis, W.J., Beach, J.A. and Berghof, O. (eds and trans.) 2006. *The Etymologies of Isidore of Seville*. Cambridge: Cambridge University Press.

Barrett, J. 2008. 'What caused the Viking Age?', *Antiquity*, 82, 671-85.

Bately, J. (ed.) 1986. *The Anglo-Saxon chronicle: MS A*. Cambridge: Brewer.

Benedictow, O. 1992. *Plague in the Late Medieval Countries*. Oslo: Middelalderforlaget.

Benedictow, O. 1996. 'Demography of the Viking Age and High Middle Ages', *Scandinavian Journal of History*, 173, 151-82.

Benedictow, O. 2004. *The Black Death*. Woodbridge: Boydell.

Biraben, J.N. and le Goff, J. 1975. 'The Plague in the Early Middle Ages', in R. Forster and P. Ranum (eds), *Biology of Man in History*, 48-80. Baltimore: Johns Hopkins University.

Bonser, W. 1963. 'Epidemics during the Anglo-Saxon Period', in W. Bonser (ed.), *The Medical Background of Anglo-Saxon England*, 51-94. London: Wellcome Historical Medical Library.

Buntrock, S. 2003. ,*Und es schrie aus den Wunden': Untersuchungen zum Schmerzphänomen und der Sprache des Schmerzes in den Íslendinga-, Konunga- und Byskupasögur sowie der Sturlunga Saga*. Unpubl. PhD, Göttingen.

Callow, C. 2006. 'Reconstructing the past in medieval Iceland', *Early Medieval Europe*, 14, 297-324.

Carniel, E. 2008. 'Plague today', *Medical History Supplement*, 27, 115-122.

Cherryson, A. 2007. 'Disturbing the dead, urbanisation, the church and the post-burial treatment of human remains in early medieval Wessex, c.600-1100AD', *Anglo-Saxon Studies in Archaeology and History*, 14, 130-142.

Clemoes, P. 1997. *Ælfric's Catholic Homilies: The First Series*. EETS S.S. 17. Oxford: OUP.

Cliff, A., Haggett, P. and Smallman-Raynor, M. 2007. 'Island epidemiology', in G. Baldacchino (ed.), *A World of Islands: An Island Studies Reader*, 267-291. Institute of Island Studies: Prince Edward Island.

Cohn, S. 2008. 'Epidemiology of the Black Death and successive waves of plague', in V. Nutton (ed.), *Pestilential Complexities*, 74-100. London: Wellcome Trust Centre for the History of Medicine.

Colgrave, B. and Mynors, R.A.B. (eds and trans.) 1969. *Bede's Ecclesiastical History of the English People*. 2nd ed. Oxford: Clarendon.

Cox, M. and Roberts, C. 2003. *Health and Disease in Britain: from Prehistory to the Present Day*. Stroud: Sutton.

Crawford, D. 2007. *Deadly Companions: How Microbes Shaped our History*. Oxford: Oxford University Press.

Crawley, R. (trans.) 1903. *The History of the Peloponnesian War, by Thucydides 431 B*. London: J.M. Dent and Co.

Creighton, C. 1965 (2nd ed.). *A History of Epidemics in Britain*, 2 vols. London: Thomas Nelson.

Dewing, H.B. (ed. and trans.) 1914-40. *Procopius with an English Translation*, 6 vols. London: Heinemann.

Diamond, J. 2006. *Collapse: How Societies Choose to Fail or Survive*. London: Penguin.

diPaolo Healey, A., Holland, J. and McDougall, D. (eds). 2007- *Dictionary of Old English A-G online*, http://tapor.library.utoronto.ca/doe/ [accessed 26/4/2010]

diPaolo Healey, A. (ed.) 2009- *Dictionary of Old English Web Corpus*. Toronto: Dictionary of Old English Project: http://tapor.library.utoronto.ca/doecorpus/

Dooley, A. 2007. 'The plague and its consequences in Ireland', in L. Little, (ed.), *Plague and the End of Antiquity: the Pandemic 541–750*, 215-28. Cambridge: Cambridge University Press.

Drancourt, M., Signoli, M., Dang, L.V., Bizot, B., Roux, V., Tzortzis, S. and Raoult, D. 2007. '*Yersinia pestis* Orientalis in remains of ancient plague patients, *Emergent Infectious Diseases*, 13/2: http://wwwnc.cdc.gov/eid/article/13/2/06-0197.htm

Dugmore, A., Keller, C. and McGovern, T. 2007. 'Norse Greenland settlement: reflections on climate change, trade, and the contrasting fates of human settlements in the North Atlantic Islands', *Arctic Anthropology*, 44, 12-36.

Duhig, C. 1998. 'The human skeletal material', in T. Malim and J. Hines (eds), *The Anglo-Saxon cemetery at Edix Hill (Barrington A), Cambridgeshire*, 154-99. York: Council for British Archaeology.

Dumville, D. and Keynes, S. (eds) 1983. *The Anglo-Saxon chronicle: a collaborative edition*. Cambridge: Brewer.

Fouracre, P. and Gerberding, R.A. (eds and trans) 1996. *Late Merovingian France: History and Hagiography 640-720*. Manchester: Manchester University Press.

Fowler, J.T. (ed. and trans.) 1894. *Adamnani Vita S. Columbae*. Oxford: Clarendon Press.

Gilchrist, R. 2008. 'Magic for the dead? The archaeology of magic in Later Medieval burials', *Medieval Archaeology*, 52, 119-168.

Grön, F. 1908. *Altnordische Heilkunde*. Harlem: De Erven.

Gräslund, B. 2007. ,Fimbulvintern, Ragnarok och klimatkrisen år 536-537 e. Kr.', *Saga och Sed*, 93-123.

Hadley, D.M. 2007. *The Vikings in England: Settlement, Society and Culture*. Manchester: Manchester University Press.

Hamerow, H. 2002. *Early Medieval Settlements: the Archaeology of Rural Communities in Northwest Europe, 400-900*. Oxford: Oxford University Press.

Hamerow, H. 2006. 'Special deposits in Anglo-Saxon settlements', *Medieval Archaeology*, 50, 1-30.

Hardy, A., Mair Charles, B. and Williams, R. 2007. *Death and Taxes: the archaeology of a Middle Saxon Estate Centre at Higham Ferrers, Northamptonshire*. Oxford: Oxford Archaeology Monograph.

Hecht, H. 1900. *Bischofs Waerferth von Worcester Übersetzung der Dialoge Gregors des Grossen über das Leben und die Wunderthaten italienischer Väter und über die Unsterblichkeit der Seelen*. Bibliothek altenglischer Prosa 5. Leipzig: G.H. Wigland.

Hennessy, W.M. and Mac Niocaill, G. (eds and trans) 2010. *Chronicon Scottorum*. Electronic edition compiled by B. Färber and R. Murphy. CELT: http://www. ucc.ie/celt/published/T100016/index.html [accessed 9/6/2010].

Hey, G. 2004. *Yarnton: Saxon and Medieval Settlement and Landscape: Results of Excavations 1990-96*. Oxford: Published for Oxford Archaeology by Oxford University School of Archaeology.

Hirst, S. and Clark, D. 2009 *Excavations at Mucking, vol. 3: The Anglo-Saxon Cemeteries*. London: Museum of London.

Howe, M. 1997. *People, Environment, Disease and Death: a Medical Geography throughout the Ages*. Cardiff: University of Wales Press.

Hufthammer, A.K. and Walløe, L. 2013. 'Rats cannot have been the intermediate hosts for *Yersinia pestis* during the medieval plague epidemics in Northern Europe', *Journal of Archaeological Science*, 40, 1752-1759.

Irvine, S. (ed.) 2004. *The Anglo-Saxon Chronicle: MS A*. Cambridge: Brewer.

Jones. T. (ed. and trans.) 1955. *Brut Y Tywysogyon* [Chronicle of Princes, Red Book of Hergest version]. Cardiff: University of Wales Press.

Jonsson, F. (ed.) 1930. *Det gamle Grönlands beskrivelse*. Copenhagen: Levin & Munksgaard.

Kaiser, C. 1998. *Krankheit und Krankheitsbewältigung in den Isländersagas: medizinhistorischer Aspekt und erzähltechnische Funktion*. Cologne: Seltmann und Hein.

Karlsson, G. 1996. 'Plague without rats: the case of fifteenth-century Iceland', *Journal of Medieval History*, 22, 263-284.

Keynes, S. 1992. 'The Comet in the Eadwine Psalter', in A. Gibson, T.H. Heslop and R. Pfaff (eds), *The Eadwine Psalter: text, image and monastic culture in twelfth-century Canterbury*, 157-164. London: Pennsylvania State University Press.

Kindschi, L (ed.) 1955. *The Latin-Old English Glossaries in Plantin-Moretus Ms 32 and British Museum Ms. Additional 32*. Ann Arbor: University Microfilms International.

Krusch, B. (ed.) 1885. *In Scriptores Rerum Merovingicarum* vol 1. Hannover: Monumenta Germaia Historica.

Krusch, B. and Levinson, W. (eds) 1951. *Gregory of Tours, History*. MGH Scriptores Rerum Merovingicarum 1.1. Hanover: Hahn.

Lee, C. 2011. 'Body talks: disease and disability in Anglo-Saxon England', in J. Roberts and L. Webster (eds), *Anglo-Saxon Traces,* 145-164. Tempe: MRTS.

Lee, C. 2011. 'Disease', in H. Hamerow, D. Hinton and S. Crawford (eds), *The Oxford Handbook of Anglo-Saxon Archaeology*, 704-723. Oxford: Oxford University Press.

Lee, C. forthcoming. 'Signs and portents: plague narratives in Icelandic sagas'. SEM 3, eds D. Banham and C. Pilsworth

Little, L. (ed.) 2007. *Plague and the end of Antiquity: the Pandemic 541–750*. Cambridge: Cambridge University Press.

Lucy, S., Tipper, J. and Dickens, A. (eds) 2009. *The Anglo-Saxon Settlement and Cemetery at Bloodmore Hill, Carlton Colville, Suffolk*. East Anglian Archaeology 131. Cambridge: Cambridge Archaeological Unit.

Lynnerup, N. 2003. 'Paleodemography of the Greenland Norse', in S. Lewis Simpson (ed.), *Vinland Revisited: the Norse World at the Turn of the First Millennium*, 133-44. St John's: Historic Association of Newfoundland and Labrador.

Mac Airt, S. (trans.) and Färber, B. (ed.) 2008. *Annals of Innisfallen*. CELT: Corpus of Electronic Texts: http://www.ucc.ie/celt/published/T100004/index.html [accessed 7/6/2010].

Mac Airt, S. and Mac Niocaill, G. (eds and trans) 1983. *Annals of Ulster*. Dublin: Institute for Advanced Studies.

McCormick, M. 2007. 'Toward a molecular history of the Justinian Pandemic', in L.K. Little (ed.), *Plague and the End of Antiquity: The Pandemic of 541–750*, 290-312. Cambridge: Cambridge University Press.

Maddicot, J. 2007. 'Plague in seventh-century England', in L. Little, (ed.), *Plague and the end of Antiquity: the pandemic 541-750*, 171-214. Cambridge: Cambridge University Press.

Mathers, D. 2009. 'A fourteenth century description of Greenland', *Saga Book* 33, 67-94.

Merritt, D. 1945. *Old English Glosses: a Collection*. MLA General Series 16. New York.

Miller, T. (ed.) 1891. *The Old English Version of Bede's Ecclesiastical History of the English People*, EETS o.s. 95, 96, 110, 111. London: Trübner.

Magner, L. 2009. *A History of Infectious Diseases and the Microbial World*. Westport: Praeger.

Montgomery, J., Evans, J.A., Powlesland, D. and Roberts, C.A. 2005. 'Continuity or colonization in Anglo-Saxon England? Isotope evidence for mobility, subsistence practice, and status at West Heslerton', *American Journal of Physical Anthropology*, 126(2), 123-38.

Morris, J. (ed. and trans.) 1980. *Nennius: British History and Welsh Annals*. Chichester: Phillimore.

Nelson, J.D. (ed. and trans.) 1991. *The Annals of St Bertin*. Manchester: Manchester University Press.

Nutton, V. (ed.) 2008. *Pestilential Complexities: Understanding Medieval Plague*. London: The Wellcome Trust Centre for the History of Medicine.

Ó Corráin, D. 1998. 'Vikings in Ireland and Scotland in the ninth century', *Peritia* 12, 296-339.

Panagiotokopulu, E., Skidmore, P., Buckland, P. and Buckland, P.C. 2007. 'Fossil insect evidence for the end of the Western Settlement in Greenland', *Naturwissenschaften*, 94, 300-306.

Price, D. and Gestsdóttir, H. 2006. 'The first settlers of Iceland: an isotopic approach to colonization', *Antiquity*, 80, 130-144.

Reff, D. 2005. *Plagues, Priests and Demons: Sacred Narratives and the rise of Christianizing the Old World and the New*. Cambridge: Cambridge University Press.

Reuter, T. 1992. *The Annals of Fulda: Ninth Century Histories*. Manchester: Manchester University Press.

Reynolds, A. 2009. *Anglo-Saxon Deviant Burial Customs*. Oxford: Oxford University Press.

Ryan, E. (ed.) and O'Donovan, J. (trans.) 2002. *Annals of the Four Masters*. CELT: Corpus of Electronic Texts: http://www.ucc.ie/celt/published/T100005A/index. html [accessed 15/12/2009].

Sallares, R. 2007. 'Ecology, evolution, and epidemiology of plague', in L. Little, (ed.), *Plague and the end of Antiquity: the pandemic 541-750*, 231-89. Cambridge: Cambridge University Press.

Samuelsson. S. 1998. *Sjúkdómar og Dánarmein Íslenskra Fornmanna*. Reykjavík: Háskólaútgáfan.

Scholz, B. and Rogers, B. (eds and trans) 1970. *Carolingian Chronicles: Royal Frankish Annals and Nithard's Histories*. Ann Arbor: University of Michigan Press.

Schuenemann, V., Bos, K., DeWitte, S., Smedes, S., Jamieson J. *et al.* 2011. 'Targeted enrichment of ancient pathogens yielding pPCP1 plasmid of *Yersinia pestis* from victims of the Black Death', *Proceedings of the National Academy of Sciences* [http://www.pnas.org/content/early/2011/08/24/1105107108; accessed 6/9/20011]

Scott, S. and Duncan, C. 2004. *Return of the Black Death: the World's Greatest Serial Killer*. Chichester: Wiley.

Shepherd-Popescu, E. (ed.) 2009. *Norwich Castle: Excavations and Historical Survey 1987-98*. 2 vols. East Anglian Archaeology 132. Norfolk: Norfolk Museums and Archaeology Service.

Signoli, M. 2012. 'Reflections on crisis burials related to past plague epidemics', *Clinical Microbiology and Infection*, 18, 218-23.

Slack, P. 1992. 'Introduction', in T. Ranger and P. Slack (eds), *Epidemics and Ideas: Essays on the Historical Perception of Pestilence*. Cambridge: Cambridge University Press.

Stephenson, J. (ed. and trans.) 1853. *History of the Kings of England: The Church Historians of England*. London: Seeleys.

Stephenson, W.H. (ed.) 1998. *Asser's Life of King Alfred*. Oxford: Clarendon.

Storm, G. (ed.) 1888. *Islandske Annaler indtil 1578*. Oslo:Christiania.

Streeter, R., Dugmore, A. and Vésteinsson, O. 2012. 'Plague and landscape resilience in premodern Iceland', *Proceedings of the National Academy of Sciences of the United States of America*, 109, 3664-3669.

Tangherlini, T. 1988. 'Ships, frogs and travelling pairs: plague legend migration in Scandinavia', *Journal of American Folklore*, 101, 176-206.

Thompson, V. 2004. *Dying and Death in Later Anglo-Saxon England*. Woodbridge: Boydell Press.

Toner, G., Fomin, M., Torma, T. and Bondarenko, G. (eds) 2007. *eDIL: Electronic Dictionary of the Irish Language*. http://www.dil.ie/index.asp.

Töpf, A. 2009. 'DNA Analysis', in E. Shepherd-Popescu (ed.), *Norwich Castle: Excavations and Historical Survey 1987-98, Vol 1*, 248-54. East Anglian Archaeology 132. Norfolk: Norfolk Museums and Archaeology Service.

Tran, T., le Forestier, C., Drancourt, M., Raoult D. and Aboudharam, G. 2011. 'Brief communication: co-detection of the *Bartonella quintana* and *Yersinia pestis* in an 11th-15th burial site in Bondy, France', *American Journal of Physical Anthropology*, 145, 489-94.

Twigg, G. 1984. *The Black Death: a Biological Reappraisal*. London: Batesford.

Waldron, T. 2007. *Paleoepidemiology: the Measure of Disease in the Human Past*. Walnut Creek: Left Coast Press.

Wiechmann, I. and Gruppe, G. 2005. 'Detection of *Yersinia pestis* in two early medieval skeletal finds from Ascheim', *American Journal of Physical Anthropology*, 126, 48-55.

Woods, D. 2004. 'Acorns, the plague and the Iona Chronicle', *Peritia*, 17/18, 495-501.

Chapter 4
The Madness of King Sigurðr: Narrating Insanity in an Old Norse Kings' Saga

Ármann Jakobsson

Illness is the night-side of life,
a more onerous citizenship.
Everyone who is born
holds dual citizenship,
in the kingdom of the well
and in the kingdom of the sick.[1]

The patient

King Sigurðr Magnússon ruled Norway for 27 years (1103–1130), first jointly with his two brothers, then with just one of them, and then finally on his own. He was one of only three out of the 18 kings who ruled Norway between 1030 and 1177 to live past the age of 35, a fact which alone would have encouraged the three kings to regard themselves as relative successes. These three kings were King Haraldr the Severe who died aged 50 in the Battle of Stamford Bridge in 1066; his son King Óláfr the Quiet who died in his bed at the age of *c.*43 in 1093; and King Sigurðr Magnússon who died aged 40 in 1130. There is some uncertainly about the age of King Eysteinn Haraldsson (d. 1157) who originally came from Ireland, whose age is never given in the extant sources and who may have lived past the age of 35, but certainly did not reach 40. It must be noted that of these three 'oldest' kings, two died natural deaths, as did several of those kings who passed away much sooner. This has to be seen in context with the inner conflicts that were a constant factor in the kingdom of Norway before 1240.[2] Before 1030, kings tended to die young as well, the exceptions being Earl Hákon Sigurðarson and his sons (who all died in their fifties as far as can be ascertained) and King Haraldr Finehair, whom it seems more appropriate to regard as a mythical rather than an actual historical figure in view of recent research;[3] indeed one of the palpably mythical aspects of King Haraldr is that he is purported to have lived into his eighties, but in the light of the rarity of any European king reaching such an age in the Middle Ages, let alone from a war-torn viking state such as 9th century Norway, and the tendency of mythical figures to live uncommonly long lives, this example can no more be taken seriously than the longevity of the biblical Methuselah. During the 13th century, the monarchy becoming stronger, Norwegian kings started living longer, including King Sverrir and King Hákon Hákonarson who lived into their late 50s.

King Sigurðr is sometimes referred to in history as *Jórsalafari*, or 'Sigurðr the Crusader', a nickname that illustrates an important fact with respect to King Sigurðr's

life and rule. Although he ruled Norway for 27 years, his reign was by defined by an event of his youth, his pilgrimage to the Holy Land during the years 1108-1111, not only by later historiography, but also by the 12th and 13th century sagas.

This study is less concerned with King Sigurðr's rule in its entirety than with his somewhat inglorious decline into madness as recounted in the 12th and 13th century Old Norse sources. The focus of this study will be on the longest account that appears in the relatively ancient kings' saga *Morkinskinna* (c. 1220), the most lengthy account of those kings of Norway who ruled between 1035 and 1157, so extensive that it must have relied on several no longer extant sources, most likely both oral and written.[4] *Morkinskinna* contains a lengthy account of Sigurðr's glorious journey to the Mediterranean wherein it is depicted as a play within a play, incorporating King Sigurðr's impersonation of a much richer, more powerful and more splendid king than he actually is. However, the saga provides not only the most extensive account of his journey, but also takes the time to expound upon his instability in later years. The juxtaposition of the two narratives demonstrates the volatility of fortune, as following the splendour of King Sigurðr's grand European tour comes the terror of his mental decline. Nevertheless, he was thought of as a successful king by both medieval and modern historiographers, his reign characterised by peace and prosperity, but followed by a succession of civil wars that lasted from 1130 to 1240.[5] This is particularly evident in Theodoricus Monachus' *Historia de antiquitate regum Norwagiensium*, wherein the authors closes his tale with Sigurðr's death because he does not want to mention the dreadful times that followed it.[6]

The narrative of King Sigurðr's madness in *Morkinskinna* is lengthy, graphic and striking. Interestingly, it is not the only account of a mental illness in this saga narrative, for the saga also includes a small anecdote about a courtier who becomes depressed and is cured by King Eysteinn, Sigurðr's brother, using a version of modern 'talk therapy' (though a couch is not mentioned).[7] In King Sigurðr's case, no therapy seems possible. His illness was clearly of the kind that defeated the combined skills of a 12th century court.

---

[1] Sontag 1978, 3.
[2] For a recent analysis of those, see Bagge 2010, esp. 23-67.
[3] See especially Á. Jakobsson 2002.

[4] See the introduction to *Íslenzk fornrit* (Aðalbjarnarson 1951, hereafter *IF*) XXIII, xxxiv-xxxix; see also Andersson and Gade 2000, 11-24.
[5] See e.g. Sigurðsson 1999, 97.
[6] Storm 1880, 67.
[7] This episode has recently been highlighted in the *British Medical Journal* by four medical experts interested in talk as therapy (Getz *et al.* 2011). See also Á. Jakobsson 2002, 151.

Below I will speak of King Sigurðr as the patient whose mental affliction caused his nearest and dearest much anxiety and chagrin. However, given that the narrative was not contemporary to his life but rather a century younger, 'King Sigurðr' must in this context refer to the character in the saga rather than the actual historical king. This article will not be much concerned with the factual accuracy of the Old Norse sources when it comes to King Sigurðr's journey. Most historians agree that King Sigurðr did arrive in Jerusalem in the summer of 1110.[8] Steven Runciman's characterisation of the Old Norse sagas as containing 'pieces of interesting historical information in the midst of legendary details' is hardly disputed either.[9] It must also be noted that characters in a given narrative do not have a will of their own, except within the artistic illusion of the narrative in question. They may thus be held to represent the author of the narrative, in this case the author of *Morkinskinna*, although the concept of saga authorship, in itself, is considerably problematic. To begin with, the identity of the author of *Morkinskinna* is not known, and it is not even certain that the saga was composed by a single author. Furthermore, there is great uncertainty as to how much of the material in the saga is original, as it is in many cases the oldest instance of a given narrative. Medieval authors did not possess their texts in the same way that modern authors do, and, when it comes to historical narrative, there is always a gap of uncertainty between the actual event and the earliest extant narrative in which it is related. In the case of King Sigurðr's golden youth and his sad decline, as depicted in *Morkinskinna*, there is a gap of some hundred years.

As will be discussed below, there is a clear link between the *Morkinskinna* narrative of King Sigurðr's madness and other prominent preoccupations of this particular text. And yet King Sigurðr is never only a saga character. Some of his energy must come from the individual who lived a century before the narrative was composed, accounts and anecdotes that must have served as the author's material for creating the King Sigurðr who appears as a character in the saga.

Youth

The scope given to the king's journey to the Holy Land in the narrative of *Morkinskinna* is a good indication of its importance within the larger framework of the history of King Sigurðr and his brothers: his crusade occupies more than a third of the narrative concerning their reign.[10] Nevertheless, its wider context, the life of King Sigurðr

as narrated in *Morkinskinna*, must be kept in mind in any analysis of the crusade account.

Before the crusade narrative begins, it is related that the three young kings were widely popular in Norway, that they reduced taxation, and that they relinquished other (un-specified) claims on their subjects.[11] It is then that King Sigurðr, out of the blue, decided to go to Jerusalem.[12] Nothing is related about the reason behind this sudden desire of his, although his aim is clearly stated: to '*kaupa sér Guðs miskunn ok góðan orðstír*' (buy himself the mercy of God and a good reputation).[13] The emphasis is placed on the great cost of the expedition and the size of his entourage. According to the poet Þórarinn Shortcloak, whose verse is used as a source in *Morkinskinna*, King Sigurðr travelled abroad with sixty ships and many magnates (landed men), although only those who were willing.[14] There seems to have been no shortage of the latter, which illustrates the glamour that a proposed journey to the Mediterranean must have held for the subjects of a peripheral monarch such as the king of Norway.

The great size of his entourage indicates that the journey was not merely a spiritual quest, but that prestige was also important to the king. Indeed, King Sigurðr's stated aims (the mercy of God and a good reputation) encompass both spiritual and cultural capital. It should thus not be overlooked that King Sigurðr must have believed that a crusade would help him after his death, and death is certainly an important subject in the earliest Norse-Icelandic biographies.[15] In King Sigurðr's case, his biography in *Morkinskinna* ends with his burial at the Church of St. Hallvarðr in Oslo and with the sentence: '*Liggr hann nú í steinveggnum útarr frá kórnum syðra [megin]*' (he now lies in the stone wall outside the choir).[16]

Whether the journey helped King Sigurðr gain his spiritual goal is a different matter. He does refer to it in the *mannjafnaðr* (flyting) with his brother Eysteinn when they compare their respective achievements,[17] but there is little emphasis here on the spiritual.[18] This flyting is a kind of spectacle, a peaceful but dramatic joust between the two kings. It also contains an evaluation of the merits of the crusade, juxtaposed with King Eysteinn's achievements at home, while he was taking care of the realm in his brother's absence. The flyting episode between the two brothers does not involve family nobility or the legitimacy

[8] See e.g. Runciman 1952, 92-93.

[9] Runciman 1952, 485.

[10] To give some indication of the scope, the text of *Morkinskinna* is 569 pages in the two volume *Íslenzk fornrit* edition. Thereof, the history of the three brothers King Sigurðr, King Eysteinn and King Óláfr occupies 82 pages, the crusade is retold in 30, thus slightly more than a third of the whole narrative. Apart from the crusade, the story of relatively friendly competition between the two brothers Sigurðr and Eysteinn is the second most consumptive narrative thread, while the insanity of King Sigurðr in later life comes third.

[11] *ÍF* XXIV, 70-71. The edition used is Jakobsson and Guðjónsson 2011. Unless otherwise stated, this article will refer to page numbers in this edition (*ÍF* XXIII and XXIV). A recent English translation of this text is Andersson and Gade 2000.

[12] Riant (1865, 175) believed that King Sigurðr had been particularly inspired by the pilgrimage of Danish king Eric (d. 1103).

[13] *ÍF* XXIV, 71.

[14] *ÍF* XXIV, 72.

[15] A case in point is the Ynglinga saga of Heimskringla, which is not so much a kings' saga but rather a collection of colourful or even downright bizarre royal deaths.

[16] *ÍF* XXIV, 152.

[17] *ÍF* XXIV, 131-34.

[18] On the flyting, see Lönnroth 1978, 53-80; Kalinke 1984, 162-65; Lie 1937, 66-68; Á. Jakobsson 2002, 183-85.

of claims to the crown, but rather the virtues, roles and obligations of a king. Sigurðr boasts of being the stronger of the two and the better swimmer, while Eysteinn claims that he is more dextrous and better at chess. Sigurðr says he is good with weapons and capable of participating in many a tournament, but people apparently turn more readily to Eysteinn to receive his judgement in their legal matters. The contest between the kings reaches its height when the achievements of the kings in office are compared. Sigurðr plays the crusade as his trump card:

> *Fór ek til Jórdánar, ok kom ek við Púl, ok sá ek þik eigi þar. Vann ek átta orrostur, ok vartu í øngarri. Fór ek til grafar Dróttins, ok sá ek þik eigi þar. Fór ek í ána, þá leið er Dróttinn fór, ok svam ek yfir, ok sá ek þik eigi þar. Ok knýtta ek þér knút, ok bíðr þín þar. Þá vann ek borgina Sídon með Jórsalakonungi, ok hǫfðum vér eigi þinn styrk eða ráð til.*[19]

(I went to Jordan and was at Apulia, and I did not see you there. I won eight battles and you were in none of them. I went to the grave of the Lord, and I did not see you there. I went to the river, by the route that the Lord took, and swam over it and I did not see you there, and I tied a knot for you that still awaits you there. Then I won the city of Sidon with the King of Jerusalem, and we did not have your support or advice.)

Eysteinn shows himself capable of fighting fire with fire and counters this with a comprehensive list of structures raised under his watch: churches, beacons, shelters, harbours, monasteries, halls and bridges. He finishes his case by mocking Sigurðr's crusade:

> *Nú er þetta smátt at telja, en eigi veit ek víst at landsbúinu gegni þetta verr eða sé óhallkvæmra en þótt þú brytjaðir blámenn fyrir inn raga karl ok hrapaðir þeim svá í helvíti.*[20]

(Now all this may not amount to much, but I am not sure that the inhabitants of the land are worse off or have profited less than when you butchered blacks for the devil and sent them to hell.)

As Sigurðr recounts his exploits on the crusade, accomplished for the glory of God, Eysteinn counters with practical achievements: the establishment of monasteries, the formulation of a body of laws, and his building enterprises, singling out merchants and fishermen amongst those who have directly benefited from his rule. Eysteinn is working for the benefit of others and is doing so in Norway. He is a king for peaceful subjects who require good roads, harbours, stable and equitable laws and monasteries. Sigurðr's crusades and courtliness are certainly remarkable, but seem in the end to be of

less practical use to his subjects in their daily lives than Eysteinn's more mundane shelters, harbours and beacons.

The flyting serves as a 'king's mirror', revealing the brothers' respective virtues and functions. Although Eysteinn proves the victor, Sigurðr's merits are obvious. But, in this episode, the crusade comes across as a fairly worldly affair: the emphasis seems to be on the cultural capital gained rather than any acquired spiritual advantage. Sigurðr does refer to Christ, but his emphasis is on the battles he has won and the places he has seen. The crusade does not seem to have made him more devout or humble. While the size of his entourage is unparalleled, his spiritual gain seems at best dubious, and it is further undermined by King Sigurðr's sad end.

The stark contrast between joy and grief lends shape to King Sigurðr the Crusader's story. In his youth he heads south and is indiscriminately received with open arms. He travels from land to land, and as he continues on the receptions become ever grander and more elaborate, the merriment more pronounced, until he finally reaches Constantinople:

> *keisari lét fara í móti þeim með leika ok sǫngfæri. Reið Sigurðr konungr ok allir hans menn með þvílíkan prís inn í borgina ok svá til halla keisara, ... þá koma þar í hǫllina tveir sendimenn Kirjalax keisara ok báru í milli sín í miklum ok stórum tǫskum bæði gull ok silfr.*[21]

(The Emperor sent out people to meet them with song and dance. King Sigurðr and all his men rode into the city in great pomp and on to the emperor's hall ... there two of Emperor Alexios's messengers entered the hall bearing huge caskets filled with gold and silver.)

In return Sigurðr holds a feast for the emperor and wins the greatest victory of many on this journey: starting a fire without wood and treating the emperor in a princely manner.

Although the Old Norse kings' sagas are clearly influenced by the ideology of divine rulership, they also emphasise charisma as an important virtue of any leader.[22] In spite of King Sigurðr's stated steadfast wish to buy himself the mercy of God, the crusade, as it is depicted in *Morkinskinna*, comes across more as an exercise in charismatic presence than as a spiritual journey. Although the matter of his salvation remains uncertain that does not necessarily imply that his wish for spiritual gain was insincere, nor that it was an unimportant part of the voyage.[23] However, it remains

---

[19] *ÍF* XXIV, 133.
[20] *ÍF* XXIV, 133-34.

[21] *ÍF* XXIV, 96.
[22] See e.g. Á. Jakobsson 1997, 89-264; Orning 2008. Orning's concepts of 'unpredictability' and 'presence' are a useful tool to illustrate the advantages (and disadvantages) that a crusade can offer to a medieval king.
[23] As Christiansen (1980, 251) has remarked, 'there is little point in trying to distinguish between crusades undertaken for pure or spiritual motives and those that were political, papalist, perverted or corrupt in

that the emphasis in the narrative of *Morkinskinna* is actually not on the spirituality of the journey, but rather on the king performing his identity successfully, and on how the crusade establishes Sigurðr as a king among kings, and Norway a kingdom among kingdoms.[24] Each royal figure that King Sigurðr meets during his voyage confers prestige on both the young king and upon his country in offering him a warm reception. Most importantly, the emperor of Constantinople entertains him with a splendid circus in the hippodrome.[25]

The splendour of King Sigurðr's magnificient journey in his youth ends up standing in stark contrast to his life at home and his sad fate later in life. The dark side of this famous journey emerges when King Sigurðr returns from his voyages - eventually in his sad fate as a lunatic on the throne, but immediately in the disruption he and his men cause upon their return. At first, King Sigurðr receives a hero's welcome, and the treasures he brings back with him cast glory on all of Norway. All hail King Sigurðr when he comes back, but soon his men start strutting around in their finery and thinking themselves above everyone who did not go on the journey, provoking a backlash from those who stayed at home. King Eysteinn's men complain that Sigurðr the Crusader's retinue consider themselves to be superior after the crusade:

> hann hefir mjǫk framizk, enda þykkir honum allt annat lítils vert, slíkt ok ǫllum mǫnnum hans, þótt þeir væri þjónostumenn í ferðinni, þá mega nú eigi jafnask við þá ríkir búendr né vinir þínir, herra. Ganga þeir nú í pellsklæðum ok hyggjask umfram margan vaskan dreng.[26]

(He has distinguished himself and he thinks everything else of little value, as do all his men as well, even if they were only his serving men on the expedition. Now neither the rich land owners nor your friends, sire, may be considered their equals, and they walk around in fur clothing and consider themselves better than many a brave man.)

The performance that earned the respect of the other kings abroad has now acquired a life of its own at home, but there it does not feel appropriate. In fact, this presages the king's own eventual sad fate.

Decline

In Constantinople, just when the king's honour is at its highest, a serpent rears its head in Paradise in the form of a prophet who spoils the happiness:

> Þat mælti spekingr einn í Miklagarði at svá myndi fara virðing Sigurðar konungs sem it óarga dýr er vaxit, geyst í bógunum ok aptr minna; lét at svá myndi fara hans konungdómr at þá myndi mest um þykkja vert en síðarr minna.[27]

(A wise man in Constantinople prophesied that Sigurðr's fame would resemble the frame of the wild beast, broad in the shoulders and tapering towards the rear; so would his kingship fare, that though at that time he was of great renown he would decline later.)

The life of a king reminds the wise man of a wild animal. Though the comparison derives from the shape of a lion, it reminds us at the same time of the animal that dwells in every civilised man.[28] King Sigurðr is now a star in the firmament, but there nevertheless dwells within him that bestial weakness which will lead to his eventual downfall.

In his youth King Sigurðr the Crusader attended a large feast surrounded by famous people. Even the emperor treated him like a brother. Later in his life he is also at a feast, but by this point everything has changed:

> Sigurðr konungr sat með mǫrgum mǫnnum gǫfgum í stirðum hug. Var þat frjákveld eitt at dróttsetinn spurði hvat til matar skyldi búa. Konungr svaraði: „Hvat nema slátr?" Svá var mikil ógn at honum at engi þorði í mót at mæla. Váru nú allir ókátir, ok bjoggusk menn til borðanna. Kómu inn sendingar ok heitt slátr á, ok váru allir menn hljóðir ok hǫrmuðu konungs mein.[29]

(King Sigurðr was sitting with many noble men in a sad state of mind. One Friday evening the steward asked what food should be prepared. The king answered: 'What else besides fresh meat?' So great was their fear of him that no one dared to contradict him. Everyone was unhappy and people prepared to eat. Steaming platters of fresh meat were borne in, and everybody was quiet and lamented the king's illness.)

The prophecy has been validated. The crusader king is now demanding to eat meat on Friday, and thereby violating Christian law. Many other stories in *Morkinskinna* dealing with the king's mental illness take place at feasts as he sits contentedly on his throne surrounded by his courtiers. The scene above recalls the king's famed progress in his youth. But Sigurðr is no longer the great monarch of old. He is now emotionally unstable, and his subjects are afraid of him. The joy of the former feast has now turned to sorrow.

The study of emotions is a relatively new subject for historians but incredibly important in studying the Middle

---

aim, execution or effect'.

[24] This has also been noted by Kalinke 1984, 155-59) who remarks: 'Sigurðr's hallmark is the grand gesture that puts him on an equal footing with the great rulers he meets' (p. 159).

[25] *ÍF* XXIV, 97-98.

[26] *ÍF* XXIV, 131.

[27] *ÍF* XXIV, 99.

[28] On lion metaphors in Old Icelandic sagas, see Beck 1972.

[29] *ÍF* XXIV, 144.

Ages, as the emotions of individuals offered an explanatory function in that period that social or economic factors absorbed in the 19th and 20th century.[30] As I have argued elsewhere, *Morkinskinna* is a saga much concerned with emotions,[31] and its narrative of King Sigurðr's decline is an excellent case study of a court governed by a mentally troubled king. As remarked by William Miller,[32] the sagas convey emotions through action and dialogue and require us to infer motivation and the emotional underpinning of human action.

At the end of King Sigurðr's story there are five episodes that reveal the king's growing disintegration.[33] In the first he is '*með miklu vanmegni ok þungu bragði... leit yfir lýðinn ok arðgaði augunum og sá umhverfis sik um pallana*' (in a bad way and extremely unhappy ... looked out over the people and rolled his eyes and looked around him at the benches).[34] The behaviour of the king is violent and only the valiant Óttarr the Trout dares to talk straight to him. Then the king calms down and agrees that he was '*œrr*' (mad).[35] On the second occasion the king is so displeased at the praise of a man as a good swimmer that he nearly drowns him,[36] and in the third incident Áslákr Rooster prevents the king from eating meat on a holy day.[37] In the fourth narrative the king is seized by lechery and yields to his weakness for meat, and in the fifth he wishes to divorce his wife and take another. In this last incident, once again a courageous subject saves the king from misfortune and the king begins to '*þrútna ok bólgna*' ('swell and puff up').[38] The symptoms are not only psychological but here become physical as well.

It is remarkable how often Sigurðr mends his ways, never punishing his subjects for preventing him from fulfilling his misguided plans, but they remain very frightened of him and at loss how to behave. On every occasion when he refuses to speak, people become afraid '*at þá myndi enn koma at honum vanstilli*' (that another attack would come over him).[39] The state of confusion that the mental illness initiates is graphically depicted in the texts, not least how baffling and terrifying the changes that come over the king appear to his court.

As his illness worsens, Sigurðr the Crusader's rule becomes a veritable reign of terror against which his subjects and his friends do not dare to protest. His insanity also leads him to various un-Christian activities such as eating meat on Fridays, abandoning his wife for another woman, and, finally, refusing to repent of his sins before his death. While *Morkinskinna* unambiguously depicts it as the result of mental illness, the king's behaviour in his later years might still seem to undo any and every spiritual advancement that he had gained with the crusade. However, the saga tends to be silent on such otherwordly matters. Although the saga demonstrates a marked interest in moral issues, it rarely speculates on the afterlife of its royal characters, and is mostly concerned with the material world.[40] *Morkinskinna* does include a prophetic narrative that could possibly be interpreted as a suggestion that King Sigurðr's place in the afterlife will be less favourable than that of his brothers, though his brother King Eysteinn offers a different interpretation, that King Sigurðr will face some serious grief in his old age, as he indeed does.[41]

Sigurðr's illness is repeatedly called *staðleysi* ('unsteadiness' or 'misplacement') or *vanstilli* ('lack of control'). In *Heimskringla* the following description occurs at the beginning of Sigurðr's illness:

> '*En er konungr var í laug ok var tjaldat yfir kerit, þá þótti honum renna fiskr í lauginni hjá sér. Þá sló á hann hlátri svá miklum, at þar fylgði staðleysi, ok kom þat síðan mjǫk optliga af honum*'

> (When the king lay in the bath and the tub was covered by a tent, he thought that fish were swimming in the bath near him. Then he began to laugh so loudly that unsteadiness followed and thereafter it happened very often to him.)[42]

In Theodoricus' *Historia*, Sigurðr is said to have been originally one of the best of rulers but later only mediocre and his madness is mentioned as having possibly been the result of a poisonous drink:

> '*Siwardus inter optimos principes tunc mertio numerandus, postmodum vero inter mediocres, dicentibus quibusdam sensum illi fuisse immutatum propter potionem cujudsam noxiæ confectionis. Sed qui hoc affirmant viderint ipsi, quid dicant; nos ista in medio relinquimus*'.[43]

The king loses his bearings and his self-control, and without self-control a king cannot be just. He is unable to discharge his responsibilities to his country and subjects. In his biography in *Morkinskinna*, this emphasis on lack of control in the king's later years is remarkably contrasted with the supreme control he demonstratesd during his performance as an excellent monarch from the North in the crusade of his youth. So the *staðleysi* is not a part of his character, it is a disease that starts afflicting him in his later days, presumably in his thirties.

---

[30] An important early study is Stearns and Stearns 1985, 813-36. The most extensive study to my knowledge is Reddy 2001, and for the Middle Ages Rosenwein 2006, who discusses some of the problems facing historians (medievalists in particular) studying emotions. As Rosenwein points out (2006, 3-5), the meaning of the word 'emotions' is far from self-evident and it could be debated whether words such as 'passions' or 'feelings' are synonymous to 'emotions', although they are used in much the same way.
[31] Á. Jakobsson 2002, 148-52.
[32] Miller 1992, 107.
[33] *ÍF* XXIV, 138-52.
[34] *ÍF* XXIV, 138-139.
[35] *ÍF* XXIV, 140.
[36] *ÍF* XXIV, 141-142.
[37] *ÍF* XXIV, 144-145.
[38] *ÍF* XXIV, 150.
[39] *IF* XXIV, 146.

[40] Á. Jakobsson 1997, 191-239.
[41] See *ÍF* XXIV, 106-8.
[42] Bjarni Aðalbjarnarson 1951, 262.
[43] Storm 1880, 66.

In the episodes concerning his madness,[44] it is clearly established how mentally unstable the king is. This is evident from the way he rolls his eyes and his erratic and unpredictable behaviour towards his wife and his subjects. The king's confused state is something that those with mentally sick relatives recognise well; the changes that come over the sick person can be baffling.

The king himself is aware of his disability. When his son, Magnús the Blind, and his alleged brother, Haraldr Gilchrist, have begun competing for power, he refers to it candidly:

> *Illa eru þér at staddir, Nóregsmenn, at hafa œran konung yfir yðr. En svá segir mér hugr um at þér mynduð rauðu gulli kaupa af stundu at ek væra heldr konungr en þeir Haraldr ok Magnús; annarr er grimmr en annarr óvitr.*[45]

(You are badly off, you Norwegians, to have a crazy king ruling you, but I suspect that you would soon pay in red gold for me to be your king rather than either Haraldr or Magnús. The first is cruel, and the other foolish.)

This evaluation proves accurate, when both men become inferior kings. Sigurðr's misfortune is of a different order: he is an excellent king who loses his mind. But his illness is not so severe as to blind him to its nature, and his sufferings in this sickness are clearly depicted.

King Sigurðr died in 1130, making these narrative accounts the only data avaible to diagnose him. Although *Morkinskinna* is quite extensive and graphic, it is still almost a century removed from the actual events. Thus it is not possible to determine what sort of mental affliction King Sigurðr suffered from, and the text provides no clue as to how it emerged. To modern medical experts, '*œrr*' (crazy) hardly suffices as a technical term and Sigurðr's unblanced behaviour could be explained by a variety of causes, physical or psychological in origin. Neither do we know how it was treated; in fact the King's subject seem more or less powerless when their ruler becomes disturbed.

What it is possible is to say is that Old Icelandic sagas demonstrate a sensitivity and an awareness of mental illnesses that today's scholarship might not expect from the 13th century North. Though the court society depicted in *Morkinskinna* offered no cure for King Sigurðr, the sympathy for his condition shines through. The madness was not explicable, and both king and subjects had to survive without those handy labels available to make people feel as if they understood what is happening.

And yet the illness of the king was still a tale worth telling and, according to the saga, the king himself remained a remarkable man in spite of his ignoble end:

> *Þat er mál manna at eigi hafi meiri skǫrungr verit né stjórnarmaðr í [Nóregi en] Sigurðr konungur. Ok þó var þat er á leið ævi hans at varla fekk hann gætt skaplyndis síns né hugar at eigi yrði þat stundum með [miklu á]felli ok þungligum hlutum. En ávallt þótti hann merkiligr konungr ok dýrligr hǫfðingi af ferð sinni ok atgervi.*[46]

(People say that there never has been a more distinguished man or ruler in [Norway than] King Sigurðr, but towards the end of his life he could hardly control his temper nor mind, so that it was not sometimes afflicted with [grave] illness and severe events, but he always was considered a remarkable king and noble ruler because of his journey and accomplishments.)

---

[44] *ÍF* XXIV, 138-152.
[45] *ÍF* XXIV, 149.

[46] *ÍF* XXIV, 131.

Bibliography

Andersson, T.M. and Gade, K.E. 2000. 'Introduction', *Morkinskinna: The Earliest Icelandic Chronicle of the Norwegian Kings (1030–1157)*. Islandica LI. Ithaca & London: Cornell University Press.

Aðalbjarnarson, B. (ed.) 1951. Heimskringla III, in *Íslenzk fornrit* XXVIII. Reykjavík: Hið íslenzka fornritafélag.

Bagge, S. 2010. *From Viking Stronghold to Christian Kingdom: State Formation in Norway, c. 900-1350*. Copenhagen: Museum Tusculanum.

Beck, H. 1972. 'Hit óarga dýr und die mittelalterliche Tiersignificatio', in J. M. Weinstock (ed.), *Saga og språk: Studies in language and literature*, 97-111. Austin: Jenkins.

Christiansen, E. 1980. *The Northern Crusades: The Baltic and the Catholic Frontier 1100-1525*. London/ Basingstoke: Macmillan.

Getz, L., Kirkengen, A. L., Pétursson, H. and Sigurðsson, J. Á. 2011. 'The royal road to healing: a bit of a saga', *British Medical Journal*, **343** (December), 7826.

Jakobsson, Á. 1997. *Í leit að konungi: Konungsmynd íslenskra konungasagna*. Reykjavík: Háskólaútgáfan.

Jakobsson, Á. 2002. *Staður í nýjum heimi: Konungasagan Morkinskinna*. Reykjavík: Háskólaútgáfan.

Jakobsson, Á. and Guðjónsson, Þ.I. (eds) 2011. Morkinskinna I-II, in *Íslenzk fornrit* XXIII–XXIV. Reykjavík: Hið íslenzka fornritafélag.

Jakobsson, S. 2002. '"Erindringen om en mægtig Personlighed": Den norsk-islandske historiske tradisjon om Harald Hårfagre i et kildekritisk perspektiv', *Historisk tidsskrift*, **81**, 213-30.

Kalinke, M.E. 1984. 'Sigurðar saga jórsalafara: the fictionalization of fact in Morkinskinna', *Scandinavian Studies*, **56**, 152-67.

Lie, H. 1937. *Studier i Heimskringlas stil: Dialogene og talene*. Oslo: Jacob Dybwad.

Lönnroth, L. 1978. *Den dubbla scenen: Muntlig diktning från Eddan till ABBA*. Stockholm: Prisma.

Miller, W. I. 1992. 'Emotions and the sagas', in G. Pálsson (ed.), *From Sagas to Society: Comparative Approaches to Early Iceland*, 89-109. Enfield Lock, Middlesex: Hisarlik Press.

Orning, H. J. 2008. *Unpredictability and presence: Norwegian kingship in the High Middle Ages*. The Northern World 38, trans. A. Crozier. Leiden/Boston: Brill.

Reddy, W.M. 2001. *The Navigation of Feeling: a Framework for the History of Emotions*. Cambridge: Cambridge University Press.

Riant, P. 1865. *Expéditions et pèlerinages des Scandinaves en terre sainte au temps des croisades*. Paris.

Rosenwein, B.H. 2006. *Emotional communities in the Early Middle Ages*. Ithaca & London: Cornell University Press.

Runciman, S. 1952. *A history of the Crusades II: The Kingdom of Jerusalem and the Frankish East 1100-1187*. Cambridge: Cambridge University Press.

Sigurðsson, J.V. 1999. *Norsk historie 800-1300: Frå høvdingemakt til konge- og kyrkjemakt*. Oslo: Norske Samlaget.

Sontag, S. 1978. *Illness as Metaphor*. New York: Farrar, Straus & Giroux.

Stearns, P.N. and Stearns, C. Z. 1985. 'Emotionology: clarifying the history of emotions and emotional standards', *American Historical Review*, **90**, 813-36.

Storm, G. (ed.) 1880. *Monumenta Historica Norvegiæ*. Kristiania (Oslo): A.W. Brøgger.

Chapter 5
'He was not an *idiota* from birth, nor is he now': false, temporary, and overturned charges of mental incapacity in 14th-century England

Wendy Turner

In November 1383, the exchequer sent an escheator to investigate whether or not Lucy Brygge of Whytechirche had been 'an *idiota* since birth'.[1] Someone informed the exchequer that she was an *idiota* and, as such, her lands 'ought to pertain to the king'. The exchequer seemed uncertain as to whether Lucy had 'fallen into such infirmity by misfortune or otherwise', but was sure she was mentally afflicted. Along with her mental state, the exchequer ordered the escheator to ascertain her age, 'the tenure and value of [her] lands', and if there were any lands that might have been sold or 'alienated' during her infirmity.[2] The escheator interviewed Lucy in mid-January 1384. Contrary to what the escheator expected, he learned that this 26 year old woman was 'not an *idiota* since her birth, nor had she fallen into any infirmity as above, but had always been sensible and of sound mind'.[3] The escheator in his reply included all of the other information that exchequer requested on the *post mortem* roll. Her lands were held of the Earl of March out of his manor of Merschwode. Lucy's holding was worth 10*s.* and were held by service of 6*d.* yearly 'and suit to the court of Merschwode twice a year'. No part of her lands had been alienated, and no other lands had descended to her.

The case of Lucy Brygge brings several questions to mind. Why was the exchequer interested in this woman's mental health? Why was the escheator handling the investigation rather than the sheriff or another royal official? Why was this investigation into the mental health of a landholder enrolled with the *post mortem* records? Most significantly, why would someone accuse a healthy woman of being an *idiota*?

A couple of the questions surrounding Lucy Brygge's case can be easily answered. By the mid-13th century, the king had established his right to collect any income from all real property held by persons born with mental conditions.[4] The crown named guardians for these persons as royal wards. For those persons who became mentally incapacitated later in life, the crown also assigned guardians and at times

collected or regulated the income from these properties, but it could not keep all the income as it could with the lands of those born mentally incompetent. Income not spent on upkeep or care was to be returned if individuals returned to health or given to their heirs when they died. In the case of Lucy, her father, Geoffrey Brygge, had held the manor of Merschwode and, presumably, the underage earl was Lucy's brother. The family manor was in the king's hands because of the heir's minority. The manor was held by knight's service and, it can be assumed, the new earl would take up his knighthood upon becoming an adult. The issue with Lucy's lands, being one of inheritance that touched upon the rights of the crown and that affected the line of inheritance for the dead earl's property, was, therefore, taken up among the *post mortem* records. This explains why the escheator was the main investigator: he was investigating a property issue. Only one question remains unanswered. Why would someone accuse Lucy, a seemingly sane woman, of mental instability?

There might be several answers to this question and, since the answer is not among the records pertaining to Lucy, other records with similar questions of mental health might provide some possible answers. In looking at other cases, it seems that the normal procedure when an heir's or landholder's mental state was in question was for the exchequer to order the escheator to confiscate all of an individual's property until the investigation was over, which was what happened to Lucy. She might have been healthy and someone was trying to tie up the inheritance proceedings for reasons of his own. Lucy might have been mentally incapacitated part of the time, having some intermittent condition that did not present at the questioning by the escheator. Lucy might have been depressed - showing signs of *melancholia* - after the death of her father from which she recovered by the time of the interrogation a few months later.[5] Yet the charge hinted at mental infirmity from birth, leaving only a few possibilities and changing the status of the income from the property in the eyes of the exchequer.

Since the crown confiscated lands of the mentally incompetent, one scenario in Lucy's case was that someone nearby thought he ought to be her guardian. No husband was mentioned in the records; therefore, Lucy was unmarried and under her father's protection until he died.[6] It seems unlikely but not improbable that a woman from a landed family would remain unmarried until 26 in the 14th century, unless something was wrong. Most

---

[1] Throughout this paper I am using the Latin *idiota* rather than the English 'idiot'. The meaning of the term 'idiot' changed over time in England, taking on negative connotations that were not present in the Middle Ages. In medieval English legal and administrative records, it is a technical term indicating a specific condition of mental health, which affected - in medieval terms - the middle or posterior of the brain and causing difficulty cogitating or remembering. For more information, see chapter 'Determining Insanity' in Turner 2013a. The quotation is found in TNA: PRO C 136/30, m 2; and CIPM v. 15, no. 908b-909, 357-8.

[2] *Ibid.*

[3] *Ibid.*

[4] For more information on royal treatment of the mentally incapacitated, see: Turner 2013a; Turner 2010a ; Turner 2013b. See also: Sutherland 1967; Clarke 1975; Roffe 2000 (accessed on 18 June 2003); Roffe and Roffe 1995 (accessed on the Internet 18 June 2003 at BMJ.com).

[5] For information on melancholia, see: Jackson 1986; 1972; Nutton 1996, 184-7; Rawcliffe 1995; Rosen 1964; Siraisi 1990; Thiher 1999.

[6] McSheffrey 2006.

women with property either took vows to the Church or married. For the time, it would be unusual to have a woman with land remain unmarried. It might be that Lucy was a widow, though her name was not listed as different from her father's. In fact, she was cited as being 'Lucy, daughter of Geoffrey atte Brygge of Whytechirche' and not 'late the wife of so-and-so'. The explanations that fit the best would be that she was sane and falsely accused by someone wanting to hold up the inheritance proceedings, or that she had same sort of intermittent mental condition with a period of lucidity at the time of the investigation.

Lucy was one among many individuals who had mysterious or unwarranted charges of mental incapacity brought against them in the 14th century. Those persons investigated for mental health reasons were normally mentally incapacitated to some degree. The crown granted mentally incapacitated landholders royal guardians to watch over them and their property. Occasionally, though, there were other reasons people appeared in the Chancery records or court cases. False charges might be levied against sane persons, individuals could have temporary insanity but were otherwise mentally healthy, charges of questioned sanity might be filed against persons with intermittent or low mental abilities, or mentally incapacitated persons returned to mental health. It is cases of sanity versus insanity - false charges, one-time charges, questionable charges, and overturned charges - that will be investigated in this paper. Since problematic mental health meant that such persons lost their abilities to make contracts, serve on juries, or other such activities involving responsibility, false accusations could freeze a person's assets, leave his neighbours in doubt as to his health and reliability, and give the crown an excuse to investigate holdings, properties, and finances. Once wardships for mentally incapacitated individuals became relatively routine in the 14th century, the idea of accusing someone of being mentally incapacitated occurred to more than one vindictive neighbour or jealous family member who took the risk of being fined in trade for having the accused financially crippled for several weeks or months.

False Charges: 'non est idiota sue'

When a landholder's mental abilities came under investigation, his life virtually stopped. His lands were confiscated, placed into protection by the crown. All land transactions were suspended, or reversed if recently made or suspected to have been made during a period in which the person might have been unable to make rational decisions. The person in question could not serve in a public capacity. He could not hold office, serve on juries, make any legal contracts, or get married. He ceased to act as a citizen and became something akin to a criminal. Sometimes arrested and held in jail, and at others allowed to wait for trial at home, these persons were treated as if already wards of the state. For example, the escheator was sent in 1383 to find out if John Bernacastell of Carlisle was 'out of his mind (*non compos mentis sue*) or not, and, if so, to take into the king's hand and keep safely until further

order all his lands, including any lands alienated by him since he went out of his mind'.[7] The escheator therefore confiscated all of John's property - even any now held by others - until the time of the trial. When interviewed, the escheator found John 'in his right mind on the day of the receipt of the above writ, and always has been'. Twelve citizens of Carlisle under oath also declared John to be sane.[8]

Once the escheator or other official found an individual sane, the escheator or a sheriff was ordered to return all the confiscated property, along with any profit that might have been made in the meantime. In another example from a 1311 close roll, Roger Wellesworth, the escheator beyond Trent, accused and later questioned John Herst. An unknown party brought it to the attention of the king that John, son of Robert Herst of Kent, might be an *idiota*. When the escheator arrived, he could not find John. The king ordered the sheriff to find John, arrest him, and bring him before the king's council at Westminster. There, John was examined, and it was 'found that he is not a madman or an *idiota*, so that his lands ought not to remain in the king's hands'.[9] Once John was known to be of sound mind, Roger was ordered to restore to John his lands and any monies collected from the lands, which had been held in the crown's custody pending the judgment on John's sanity. William Maureward, in another case, also had all his property restored to him once he was discovered to be sane. In December 1308, 'William Maureward was examined before the king's council at Westminster, whom Ralph Basset had arrested by the king's writ as a madman and an *idiota*, and it is found that he is not a madman and an *idiota*, but is wise and sufficient for the government of his affairs, and so he is dismissed'.[10]

There were other cases of false accusations. One peculiar issue is that the accuser was rarely named, and all accusations involving property seem to be investigated. Who could blame the king or exchequer? There was money to be made if a person became a ward of the crown. Even when the accuser includes his name, the accusation is often in terms of hearsay, so that the accuser cannot be held liable if the accusation is proved false. When John Besevill was accused in 1380, the exchequer sent the escheator in May 'to enquire concerning a report that the said John son of John is an *idiota*'. In June, the escheator wrote back that 'the said John son of John is not, and never has been, an *idiota*'.[11] Hamo Waltham, who was accused in 1362, demonstrates how the king could profit from wardship. While Hamo Waltham's lands were under the king's jurisdiction, pending trial, and since Hamo was supposedly an *idiota*, the king presented Denis Lopham with the gift of the church of Staynyngchurch in November

---

[7] TNA: PRO C 136/29, m 12; CIPM v. 15, no. 894b-895 (p. 353).
[8] For information on how the law worked, see especially: Green 1985; Brand 1992; Palmer 1993; 1982.
[9] TNA: PRO C 54/129, m 30; CCR 1307-1313, 367.
[10] TNA: PRO C 54/126, m 17d - (cancelled); CCR 1307-1313, 132. See also: TNA: PRO C 260/13, no 6 and C 262/5, no 2.
[11] TNA: PRO C 136/11, m 6; CIPM v. 15, no. 289/90, 117.

1362.[12] During a wardship, the king not only assigned the mentally incapacitated person a guardian, but could also name all officials to church offices. A month later, the king had to revoke the presentation because he 'was deceived' in the assumption that Hamo was mentally incompetent: 'Hamo is not an *idiota* and his lands are not in the king's hands'.[13] When Joan Hayme was accused in 1393, the exchequer sent a commission of three men to question Joan, 'late the wife of Richard Hayme', because she had been reported to be 'an *idiota* of unsound mind'.[14] The commissioners - Robert Whityngton, Thomas Walweyn, and Thomas Brugge - along with the sheriff of Gloucester were to discover if the report on Joan Hayme was true. As well, they were to find out for how long she had been in a state of idiocy, whether she had times of lucidity, and what lands belonged to her and if they were held in service. Later that year, the commission responded to the charges, writing: 'The said Joan has never been an *idiota*, nor is she one at present. From the earliest age she has been of sound mind, and still is'. Here again, Joan seems not to be an *idiota* in any way; quite the contrary, she had a 'sound mind', according to this record, but again, like Lucy, Joan had no male to protect her and someone might have wanted to push her aside in favor of a male heir. This does not mean that more women were falsely accused though: most individuals falsely accused of mental incapacity were men, which was statistically because most landholders were men.

One-Time Charges: Temporary Insanity

Medieval English administrators, as well as physicians, knew the difference between those persons with epilepsy or another illness and those with a mental incompetence or disability.[15] For example, in July 1299, the escheator was to find out the state of John Romesye, who was reported to be an *idiota*, possibly from birth. The escheator found that 'the said John had been of sound mind from his birth until now, but when he was 15 he fell into a falling sickness'.[16] This same record rehearses some of his important land transactions, such as when he was 24 and enfeoffed Alan Plogenet and his heirs with all of his lands in Modyford Terry. Records of this type often state that the accused 'was then of sound mind', so that there would be no questioning of the person's mental state at the time of the legal transaction.

Other persons became mentally impaired while ill, lashing out at persons near them or those trying to help them. The administrators were quite clear in their distinctions between the mentally incapacitated and those sane persons who are

ill. The persons in these records were normally quite sane, but while physically ill they demonstrated lapses in mental health for one reason or another - a high fever, extreme pain, acute disease, etc. Because these cases involve sane persons committing abuse or murder, they were often reported in court records as criminals, rather than in land records or administrative accounts. Four brief cases will provide some idea of the types of temporary insanity that normally rational persons underwent in medieval England. Gilla (Guillaume?) Blackburn killed Amoria, his wife, 'while ill with that of madness ... raving (*in infirmitas illa amens [...] furiosus*)'.[17] Gilla was ill (*infirmitas*) and became demented (*amens*) to the point of not understanding his actions, and he in fury (*furiosus*) murdered his wife. Another man, Thomas le Hest, murdered his son Stephen when he was ill (*infimitate*). His illness brought on frenzy and while he was frenzied (*in frenesiam*), he killed his son.[18] John Beneit of Wodenese murdered his wife and two daughters. John was ill, when he 'became frenzied, while laboring under acute disease (*per frenesimus morba acute labortas*)', and destroyed the lives of his family.[19] Nicholas Stut of Bray was also ill (*infirmitate*) and became frenzied (*frenesi*).[20] He killed a neighbor, Isabella, the wife of Peter Pyrye. Most of those persons with temporary insanity who lashed out and murdered killed someone close to them; Gilla killed his wife, Thomas his son, John his wife and daughters, and Nicholas a neighbour. Whether their stories were true is not the point; rather the significance lies in the wording of the records, that each was ill and became frenzied (*frenesis*) or raging (*furiosus*). This was the turning point for a jury; if the guilty party had no intent to harm, he should not be punished for his actions.

All of these men were pardoned for the crime of homicide because of their temporary states of insanity. Each had to prove in some way that he had been mentally incapacitated at the time of his crime, either with witnesses to his illness, testimony as to the shock he was in after the fact, or some evidence of the illness out of which his frenzied or raging state arose. The information guiding judges and juries was in part formulaic, which is why all of these cases sound so similar in format and substance. The testimony did not exonerate these men of their guilt in the crime of homicide, but could pardon them from punishment.[21]

Questionable Charges: Checking and Rechecking

When Lucy was questioned, the escheator probably used a standard set of questions to test an individual's memory, cognitive abilities, and understanding. For example, the exchequer sent the escheator in May of 1341 to examine Thomas Grenestede 'personally' and find out 'whether he is an *idiota*, as is said, or not'.[22] The escheator wrote

---

[12] TNA: PRO C 66/266, m 16; CPR 1361-1364, 264.
[13] Listed here as 'Hamonis': TNA: PRO C 66/266, m 5; CPR 1361-1364, 277.
[14] TNA: PRO C 136/79, m 11; CIPM v. 17, no. 276, 124-5.
[15] The term 'disability' was not used in the Middle Ages. Yet, the concept that someone was impaired to the point of needing assistance or being unable to work was evident. Therefore, not all persons who were mentally incompetent were disabled - needing a guardian. For more general information on the term 'disability,' see: Metzler 2006.
[16] TNA: PRO C 133/92, m 4; CIPM v. 3, no. 548, 423.

[17] TNA: PRO JUST 1/422, m 1d.
[18] TNA: PRO C 260/4, no 13b.
[19] TNA: PRO C 66/109, m 6. See also: CPR 1281-1292, 390.
[20] TNA: PRO C 66/134, m 4; C 260/21, no 10b; C 260/3, no 19; and CPR 1307-1313, 304.
[21] Waugh 1988, 115; Butler 2007, 214-215.
[22] TNA: PRO C 135/65, m 20; CIPM v. 8, no. 340, 236.

that he went to Horsham 'in the neighbourhood of West Grenestede' but could not find Thomas. He asked the neighbors their opinions of Thomas, collecting their testimony, and a few days later interviewed Thomas himself. The escheator 'found [Thomas] of good mind and sane memory in word and deed, counting money, measuring cloth and doing all other things'.[23] Escheators regularly used such common activities as giving directions, measuring, recalling names of family members, or making change. The escheator seemed to have some doubt about Thomas and returned in June and again in October to check on him. Each time the escheator wrote to the exchequer that he found Thomas 'of good, clear, and sound memory, and always was from his birth'.[24] Thomas was the heir of his father Griffin Grenestede, and held his lands from John Moubray; his property was small but not insignificant. Yet, Thomas Grenestede had paid his fine in the king's court to alienate some of his lands to John Humeri, which might have touched off the initial investigation. It might have appeared odd to have so easily parted with an inheritance. Given the number of times Thomas was questioned, he or someone close to him must have said or done something that placed doubt in the mind of the escheator. Perhaps Thomas had an intermittent condition, which would be hard to document.

An individual did not have to be of high intelligence to be 'sane', rather he had to be aware and competent enough to carry out his responsibilities in his property, in his community, and to his king and country.[25] When the escheator was in doubt as the competence of an individual, he could and did question relatives and neighbours. If doubt remained, the escheator could send the individual to the exchequer, the king's council, parliament, or even the king. For example, the escheator, Walter Goucestria, was asked in July 1305 to inquire 'whether the king can give the wardship of the lands which ought to descend to [Peter Champeneys] in Soterton to whom he pleases etc. or not'. The son and heir of John Champeneys, Peter inherited a messuage held of the abbot of Croyland, 54 acres of arable land held from various persons, seven acres of meadow, and over six acres of pasture and another six of marsh. All totalled, Peter held a patchwork of 74 acres and a messuage. The escheator investigated the state of Peter finding him 'not an *idiota*, so that the king cannot give the wardship of him or his lands to anyone to his prejudice'.[26] But there was doubt, so Peter was sent forward to the king's council to be examined, and they, too, found him to be 'not an *idiota*'. They commanded the escheator to restore Peter's lands 'together with everything received thence since they were taken into the king's hands'.[27] The crown did not want people thinking that he falsely took away lands from sane individuals. He wanted to be absolutely sure, or at least to have no questions raised, about those lands from which he would ultimately make a profit.

Questionable Charges: Aging as Mental Incapacity

It was one thing for the crown to confiscate the lands of a young individual with obvious mental health problems. It was another to strip an elderly person, who served the crown or community well for decades, and who now - in retirement - found he or she was having trouble with memory or cognition. Yet, relatives and neighbours sometimes legally questioned odd choices in wills written in the last years or days of life. For example, ten days before he died in 1305, Ralph Pyrot granted the manors of Sauston and Lyndesle to his younger son Simon for life. Simon had custody the manors for only 15 days, when the escheator took them into the king's hand. These lands were held of the king in chief for two knight's fees, doing the service of one knight in war. A question arose concerning the sanity of Ralph senior on his deathbed, since his heir was his 13-year-old grandson, Ralph, son of Ralph senior's eldest son, also named Ralph, and not Simon. Did Simon manipulate his father into allowing him these manors for life at a time in which his father may not have had his full mental faculties? Through witnesses the escheator learned that Ralph senior was 'sound in will and memory (*in bona voluntate et memoria*)'[28] when he gave the property to Simon. Though the escheator reports this as truth, there remains a possibility that the witnesses lied to help Simon. Nevertheless, the law stated that insanity could not be proved after death. In other words, unless the insanity was 'known' before hand and it was unquestionably Ralph's state of mind, the escheator would have found him sane and the transaction valid.[29]

It was not uncommon for wills to be questioned or contested, and sometimes the questions revolved around doubts about the mental health of the one making the will, especially if changes were made at the last minute. This concept went hand-in-hand with doubts about the mental competence of older people. As a person aged, certainly he might have a loss of his mental sharpness, but that did not necessarily make him mentally incapacitated. Royal officials investigating the elderly made this sort of distinction. For instance, the escheator examined the 60-year-old William Venour, 'an *idiota* as the king has heard', in October 1328. The escheator found William 'sufficiently discreet', but inquired into the matter in any case because he wanted to alleviate any doubt.[30] By February 1329, the escheator became convinced that 'William was not an *idiota* at his birth, nor has been up to this time'. William held a toft and a one-acre meadow from the bishop of Chester for 5*s*. 8*d*. yearly. The inherited lands were in the hands of Hugh Rider, most likely the man charged with caring for them until the date of the trial. Though no release of the lands was stated here, it would have been sent either to the local sheriff or to the escheator within a month or so, since there was nothing wrong with William.

[23] TNA: PRO C 135/63, m 8; CIPM v. 8, no 284, 209.
[24] CIPM v. 8, no. 340, 236 and no. 284, 209.
[25] Clark 1994. See also: Rosen 1964, 377-388.
[26] TNA: PRO C 133/120, m 4; CIPM v. 4, no. 326, 222-3; Rubin 1987.
[27] TNA: PRO C 54/122, m 3; CCR 1305-1307, 299.

[28] TNA: PRO C 133/120, m 3; CIPM v. 4, no. 325, 222.
[29] See below, note 36.
[30] TNA: PRO C 135/14, m 7; CIPM v. 7, no. 181, 148.

At other times, escheators found aging landholders being taken advantage of because of their deficient mental abilities. Yet, most of the time, aging landlords were treated under the law as if sane with temporary mental health issues. In the late 13th century, William Percy of Kildale was just such a man. Two inquisitors, John Reygate and Geoffrey Aguyllun, questioned William and his family and neighbours, while William sat, emotionally overwrought, weeping at the hearing.[31] William could not remember having granted to his son the manor of Kildale, from which his son seems to have barred William. William wanted to go home and practically begged the inquisitors to allow him to do so. William had dispersed other properties, manors and lands, to his several sons and to the neighbours. Yet, at the trial, he had no memory of these events. The inquisitors' judgment was that William had become 'wholly impotent of body and not of sound mind'.[32] Even the wording here is to safeguard the crown against any question that kept William from his rightful property. The inquisitors had two choices: they could treat William as sane with temporary insanity on the day of the hearing - which meant that his transactions would stand; or, they could say he was mentally disabled and confiscate his property and assign him a guardian. The second would void his transactions with his sons. Many issues would have to be considered before creating such chaos in many lives - how long ago did he grant them? Was a legal document drawn up at the time? If so, there was precedent for trusting earlier judges to have accounted for mental health before proceeding with land transactions.

In another variation on this theme, Eustacia Heselarton seemed to have been quite aware, or at least aware enough to ask for help before she found herself in William's position. Eustacia was the daughter and heir of Peter Percy from whom she inherited while she was underage. Her guardian as a child was Geoffrey Scrop. At some point, she married Walter Heselarton.[33] In 1327, her husband pressed the crown to release her lands into his control when she came of age.[34] By 1350, Eustacia was a widow. At that time, and quite unusually, she petitioned the crown for a guardian. The petition explained 'that she is now broken by age and very feeble, and on that pretext grievances and injuries are done to her daily and her lands, which are held in chief, and goods are destroyed in many ways'. Eustacia must have been in her early 40s when she wrote that she was 'broken by age and very feeble,' and exactly why she would use these words is hard to explain. Perhaps she was simply a sickly person, or had lingering complications from childbirth, or felt lost without a male protector. Or, perhaps she had a mental health issue, becoming forgetful or lost; the petition does not explain.

The king 'for her greater security' granted her the requested assistance in the form of guardians 'and defenders of her and her lands during her pleasure'. These three men, Thomas Ughtred, John Hothum of Scoreburgh the younger, and Martin Skiryn, clerk, supported her out of her estate and answered 'to her for any balance left over'.[35] This gave Eustacia some power in the relationship between her and her guardians. They certainly must have met her at some point, which was one reason the king may have had doubts as to Eustacia's mental condition later. If Eustacia showed signs of mental incompetence, her guardians should have reported it. Nevertheless, in 1367, when her son Walter came of age to inherit, she was listed as 'an *idiota* from birth as the jurors were informed'. This record must have been written shortly after her death because it continues on to explain that 'because idiocy may not by the law and custom of the realm be proved and examined after the death of the *idiota*',[36] the king would have to drop any claim on the profits from the lands. In other words, if she had been an *idiota a nativite*, incompetent from birth, the crown would have been able to keep the profits from the land. But, because she had only been in the king's custody as an feeble individual - in body, not mind - the king would have to return all profits to the heir, Walter, since 'the king considers the cause of taking [the income] into his hand insufficient'.[37] It was almost as if the king could tell that information was being withheld from him, and that the three guardians - Thomas Ughtred, John Hothum, and Martin Skiryn - all knew the truth of the matter, but were not saying.

It is remarkable how many cases come up where the king does not press a matter to his own advantage. He wanted to appear to be within the law at all times.[38] In cases of confusion in aged individuals, they were treated as if temporarily mentally incapacitated. Someone was paid out of the estate to care for them and a legal guardian made certain that their property was protected. There was abuse of the system, of course, but on the whole it worked well.[39] There were steps in place to make sure the individual got a fair hearing. Questionable cases could be handed over to higher authorities, such as the exchequer or the king's council, and cases could be appealed. Like all such matters, this favoured those who could afford the legal fees, but there were checks in the system. The crown did not want someone stripped of his lands, unless he was most definitely mentally incapacitated.

Overturned Charges: Intermittent Sanity

Under certain circumstances charges of mental incapacity were overturned and all royal involvement with the individual and his household was withdrawn. As shown

---

[31] This paper has a couple of very late 13th century documents. The title should have been the 'long-14th century.' This case is from 1285. It is a good example of a landlord who had lost his power of reason and was confused at the hearing, I could not leave it out. I have taken up this case in more detail elsewhere: Turner 2010b.

[32] TNA: PRO C 133/42, m 14; CIPM v. 2, no. 584.

[33] CIPM v. 7, no. 622, see especially, 421.

[34] CIPM v. 8, no. 705, 515.

[35] TNA: PRO C 66/232, m 4; CPR 1350-1354, 19

[36] TNA: PRO C 54/205, m 15; CCR 1364-1368, 340.

[37] TNA: PRO C 54/205, m 15; CCR 1364-1368, 340.

[38] For more on law generally, and those works that have influenced my statements here, see: Biancalana 2001; Bothwell 2004; Brand 1994; Lyon 1980; Palmer 1993; 1982; Waugh 1991; 1988.

[39] Turner, 'Guardians,' chapter in 2013a.

above, when an individual's mental capacity was challenged, his lands were taken into the king's hand and held pending the hearing of whether or not the person was sane. When the individual in question was found to be capable, the crown released the person's property back into his care. The same was true of those mentally incapacitated persons who had intermittent sanity. They would have difficulty for a while, then be completely sane and intelligent later. When difficulty was reported, the crown stepped in and assigned him a guardian. When the individual was once again healthy, his lands were returned to him. At least, that was how it was supposed to work. Some guardians became dependent upon their stipends as guardian and would not report their wards' return to health. If this happened, a mentally incapacitated person, who was no longer incapacitated, would often turn to relatives or friends to go to court for him, since that privilege was revoked for all mentally incapacitated persons.

As was suggested in the case of Lucy Brygge, neighbours or relatives might falsely report mental incompetence for selfish reasons - either they wanted a chance to become the guardian of the property, or out of spite they wished to keep a person from jury service or other office. For example, in April 1300, the escheator headed out to Helleston to inquire after the manor of Trelewyth and the hamlets of Treworien, Polgrun, and Bagahenele, all of which were part of Ralph Trelewith's estate. The escheator questioned his neighbours, who reported that Ralph 'has been such an *idiota* and mentally incompetent from his birth (*idiota & non compos mentis sue a nativitate*) until now that he cannot manage his affairs.'[40] Ralph was not at home when the escheator went to see him in person; later when Ralph was questioned, the chancellor reversed the escheator's decision. 'Ralph having appeared in person before the chancellor at Lincoln, and being examined, was found to be sane and fit to manage his own affairs.'[41] This seems to have begun as a normal *post mortem* investigation upon the death of Ralph's father, Richard, with no explanation given as to why the neighbours thought Ralph was mentally incompetent.

Roger Stanlake and John Brewes were both mentally incapacitated at times. The question was never 'do they have problems managing their estates?' The obvious answer was 'sometimes.' The real question was, 'when do they need assistance and when not?' They were both given guardians, but the push and pull between wanting independence and having a guardian became expensive and problematic for the mentally afflicted men, their families, and the crown.

Roger Stanlake had an intermittent condition. At first, in December 1373, Roger appeared to have been falsely accused and John Froille, the escheator, was 'order[ed] to remove the king's hand, and not to meddle further with the lands of Roger son of Richard de Stanlak, delivering

up any issues thereof taken; as lately upon information received that the said Roger was an *idiota* from birth (*idiota a nativitate*) so that he was not capable of ruling himself or his lands...'[42] The escheator questioned 'true men' in the surrounding area as to the state of Roger, 'an *idiota* or no?' At the next court date, the chancellor and the king's justices at Westminster examined Roger. They decided 'he was of sound mind, capable of ruling himself and his lands, and not an *idiota*.' All of his property was returned to him, which the crown officials had held pending the trial. There was doubt from the beginning and Roger was reexamined periodically as to his state by commissions or escheators. In 1365, a commission of three men labelled Roger 'fatuous and an *idiota* (*fatuus et idiota existit*) so that he is insufficient for the rule of himself and his lands and goods.'[43] In 1373, the escheator investigated and found that, after several accusations of alienation of lands and idiocy, 'Roger was not an *idiota* from birth; nor is he now. He was born at Wytteneye and brought up there until he was 15 years of age. He went to school there, and was well able to read before he left.'[44] In 1377, the escheator Nicholas Somerton found him 'an *idiota* from birth.'[45] In 1399, this finding was confirmed when an inquiry was sent to see if Roger was still a '*mere fatuus et idiota.*' They found him in the same '*ignorant*' condition.[46] The overall picture of Roger was that of an intelligent individual who had an intermittent mental condition of some type that periodically kept him from being able to function in medieval English society.

John Brewes also had an intermittent condition, so that he was able to marry and have children. John and his wife were in and out of court over the years, much like Roger. John had three guardians for his various properties, having been found an *idiota* on several occasions. At times, though, John would be better and his lands would be returned to him and his wife. In June 1361, John was 'found no *idiota* (*Brewosa* [...] *idiota non est*),'[47] and his lands were returned to him. But four years later, John was again named an *idiota* when the king presented John Aleyn of Huntyngdon to the church of Wauton, one of John's responsibilities.[48] In 1368, the escheator described John as 'an *idiota* from his birth and [he] enjoys no lucid intervals,'[49] even though earlier he had been found sane before the council on a couple of occasions. He had to have been sane at the time of his marriage as well. It was true that upon occasion a few mentally incapacitated persons without lucid intervals were married off, even though that was forbidden; yet, once together, it was also frowned upon to pull them apart. John, though, since he was known to have sane periods, probably married during a time of lucidity.

---

40 TNA: PRO C 133/98, m 9 and CIPM v. 3, no. 614, 492.
41 See CIPM v. 3, no. 614, 492.

42 TNA: PRO C 54/211, m 5; CCR 1369-1374, 526.
43 TNA: PRO C 66/272, m 25d; CPR 1364-1367, 202.
44 TNA: PRO C 135/235, m 13; CIPM v. 13, no. 269, 264-5.
45 TNA: PRO C 145/212, no 11; CIM v. 4, no. 11, 6.
46 TNA: PRO C 137/19, m 89; CIPM v. 18, no. 318, 103.
47 TNA: PRO C 54/199, m 24d and m 26; CCR 1360-1364, 189 and 273-4.
48 TNA: PRO C 66/271, m 37; CPR 1364-1367, 82.
49 TNA: PRO C 135/204, m 13; CIPM v. 12, no. 271, 255.

Illness or stress played a part in John Berton's quite different story. He seems to have had problems after the death of his father. In 1345, John briefly had a guardian, Thomas Mussenden (or Missynden), when the charge of being an *idiota* was reversed by the Chancery.[50] Something happened then - either Thomas refused to give up the guardianship or convinced everyone, including the escheator, Thomas Aspale, that John was indeed an '*idiota and madman*' (*idiota et non compos mentis sue*). Nine years later, Thomas Aspale, no longer serving as escheator, was called back to testify. Thomas Aspale reported that John had been 'an *idiota*[51] for sixteen years, always in the same state without lucid intervals [... and that he had] committed the keeping of [John's properties] to Thomas de Mussenden'.[52] John had somehow brought suit against Mussenden and his wife Isabel, 'suggesting that he was of sound mind and had been so at the time of the taking of the inquisition and before, and praying for restitution of this lands, with the issues thereof while in [the] king's hands.'[53] In the same report, the king ordered Thomas Aspale to re-examine the case and, moreover, to find the truth of the matter by 'personal examination as well as by the inquisition'. Thomas did this and John's statement is most illuminating. John reported that,

> [F]rom his infancy until his completion of the age of twenty-one years and more was of sound mind (*compos mentis*), having no kind of idiocy, but, because of a great fright and excessive grief (*ex maximo terore et nimius tristioia* [sic]) because of his father's death, he afterwards sustained almost total loss of memory and remained in that state for three years, although with occasional lucid intervals, after which he recovered and his memory was restored and remained so for more than five years before the date of the said inquisition.[54]

What exactly had happened to John cannot be known for certain, but since his father's death was only a couple of years before the Black Death, he might have been in shock at all the death around him, prolonging his condition. John's lands were restored to him with all the profits after the hearing in 1345, except one manor. Most often when an individual became mentally afflicted later in life, the crown gave his wardship to a family member. Although this is not expressed directly, the crown makes an interesting provision for Thomas Mussenden and his wife Isabel, who is most likely John's heir (sister?). The king explained that he did not want any prejudice held against Mussenden, his wife, or their heirs later because of idiocy alleged against John - implying that they would inherit John's properties. To that end, the king gifted Mussenden and his family with the manor of Farle and the advowson of the church in the town, 'which Mary late the wife of James atte Berton

[John's father] held in dower of the inheritance of the said John'.[55] This lessened John's holdings, and the change in the inheritance line is not explained.

Conclusion

Some sane persons demonstrated characteristics of mental incapacity and were accused of being mentally incapacitated. Evidence of a false accusation or a return to sanity, either because it was temporary or intermittent, could lead the crown to withdraw or dismiss charges of mental incapacity. If a sane person committed a crime while ill and there was evidence to believe that this sane individual might have been insane for a moment, the punishment was most often lifted. Persons with questionable mental health conditions or known recurrent afflictions were re-examined periodically as to their mental state. They were otherwise allowed all the normal privileges of any sane person. All of these royal administrative actions were an attempt by the crown to keep the public safe and in particular, as these examples show, landholders and their inheritances.

More important to this study are those cases of false accusation. Lucy Brygge of Whytechirche was just one person who had false charges of mental incapacity brought against her. As seen in the other cases and circumstances outlined here, a report or a question concerning an individual's mental competence could be brought up by anyone, as in the case of Simon Pyrot, whose father, Ralph, came under scrutiny. Ralph's will and sanity were questioned since, only days before he died, Ralph gave Simon lands out of the general inheritance, even if only for life. Lucy was in a similar situation since her father had left her lands out of his estate, lands which would normally have descended to her younger brother. Since her father was the former earl of March, it was not likely that his mental health could be questioned, so it was Lucy - a single, now unprotected female - who had her mental competency under review. Furthermore, as in the records of Eustacia Heselarton, whose mental health was suspect after her death, the officials wrote that 'because idiocy may not by the law and custom of the realm be proved and examined after the death of the *idiota*',[56] the king could not retroactively claim Eustacia to have been an *idiota a nativitate* (from birth). Lucy's father, therefore, could not have been questioned as to the state of his mental health in any case, and anyone concerned with her gaining at her brother's expense would have to find another avenue to pursue the matter.

Although hypothetical, it is worth pondering, if only to find new paths for research, who would have wanted to change Lucy's inheritance? Who would second-guess her father's intent when he portioned off a small part of his estate from his under-aged son's inheritance for his adult, unmarried daughter? One who might have filed the complaint against

---

[50] TNA: PRO C 60/145, m 30–(cancelled); *CFR* v. 5, 410-411.
[51] Elsewhere in this record, John was referred to as '*idiota et fatuitatis.*' TNA: PRO C 66/242, m 7.
[52] TNA: PRO C 66/242, m 7; CPR 1354-1358, 44-45.
[53] *Ibid.*
[54] *Ibid.*
[55] *Ibid.*
[56] TNA: PRO C 54/205, m 15; CCR 1364-1368, 340.

Lucy would be the guardian of the young earl, Lucy's brother. The guardian was supposed to be looking out for the estate of the earl of March, not overseeing the best interest for all the former earl's children. Any division of the property might have looked suspicious. And one way to quickly hold up the transfer of property out of the estate at large was to accuse the receiving party of mental incompetence.

The case of Lucy Brygge demonstrates above all that the English administrative system whenever possible looked out for those accused of mental incompetence, those inheriting property underage, and the wishes of a dead father. Lucy would have been asked a standard set of questions at a hearing, most likely by the escheator. Those questions would have covered her ability to perceive the world around her, to understand what she perceived, and to remember it. The escheator, much as he did with Thomas Grenestede, would have asked Lucy common questions about making change, measuring cloth, and recalling the names of family members. Once her mental capacity was proved to the satisfaction of the escheator, her lands would have been returned to her by the exchequer or crown. If there were a question about her mental state, the escheator could have sent her to be questioned by the exchequer, the king's council, justices, or the king. If found mentally incompetent, Lucy would have been given a guardian and the guardian and crown would then be responsible for the property her father had left her. And, if she were found competent, the crown would return her lands. Either way, the lands were hers and could not be contested. Lucy Brygge was a landholder and heir, and most likely falsely accused of being an *idiota*.

Bibliography

Biancalana, J. 2001. *The Fee Tail and the Common Recovery in Medieval England, 1176-1502*, Cambridge Studies in Legal History, Cambridge: Cambridge University Press.

Bothwell, J.S. 2004. *Edward III and the English Peerage: Royal Patronage, Social Mobility and Political control in 14th-Century England*, Woodbridge: Boydell.

Brand, P.A. 1992. *The Making of the Common Law*, London & Rio Grande: The Hambledon Press.

Butler, S.M. 2007. *The Language of Abuse: Marital Violence in Later Medieval England*, Leiden and Boston: Brill.

CIPM - 1904-1970. *Calendar of Inquisitions Post Mortem and other Analogous Documents Preserved in the Public Record Office*, Public Record Office, 20 vols. London: HMSO.

CIM - 1916-1968. *Calendar of Inquisitions Miscellani (Chancery), Henry III-Henry V*, Public Record Office, 7 vols. London: HMSO.

CCR - 1892-1954. *Calendar of the Close Rolls Preserved in the Public Record Office, 1227-1485*, Public Record Office. 45 vols. London: HMSO.

CPR - 1891-1901. *Calendar of the Patent Rolls Preserved in the Public Record Office, 1216-1509*, Public Record Office, 52 vols. London: HMSO.

Clarke, B. 1975. *Mental Disorder in Earlier Britain: Exploratory Studies*, Cardiff: University of Wales Press.

Clark, E. 1994. 'Social welfare and mutual aid in the medieval countryside', *Journal of British Studies*, **33**, 381-406.

Green, T.A. 1985. *Verdict according to Conscience: Perspectives on the English Criminal Trial Jury, 1200-1800*, Chicago & London: University of Chicago Press.

Hudson, J. 1994. *Land, Law, and Lordship in Anglo-Norman England*, Oxford: Clarendon Press.

Jackson, S.W. 1986. *Melancholia and Depression from Hippocratic Times to Modern Times*, New Haven and London: Yale University Press.

Jackson, S.W. 1972. 'Unusual mental states in Medieval Europe: I. medical syndromes of mental disorder, 400-1100 AD', *Journal of the History of Medicine and Allied Sciences*, **27/3**, 262-297.

Lyon, B. 1960 (2nd ed. 1980). *A Constitutional and Legal History of Medieval England*, New York & London: W.W. Norton.

McSheffrey, S. 2006. *Marriage, Sex, and Civic Culture in Late Medieval London*, Philadelphia: University of Pennsylvania Press.

Metzler, I., 2006. *Disability in Medieval Europe: Thinking about Physical Impairment during the High Middle Ages c. 1100 – 1400*, London: Routledge.

Nutton, V. 1996. 'Medicine in Medieval Western Europe', in L.I. Conrad *et al.*, (eds), *The Western Medical Tradition 800 BC to AD 1800*, Members of the Academic Unit: The Wellcome Institute for the History of Medicine London, 139-198. Cambridge: Cambridge University Press.

Palmer, R.C. 1993. *English Law in the Age of the Black Death, 1348-1381: A Transformation of Governance and Law*, Chapel Hill & London: The University of North Carolina Press.

Palmer, R.C. 1982. *The County Courts of Medieval England 1150-1350*, Princeton, NJ: Princeton University Press.

Rawcliffe, C. 1995. *Medicine and Society in Later Medieval England*, London: Sandpiper Books.

Roffe, D. 2000. 'Perceptions of insanity in medieval England,' *Body and Mind Seminar, Department of Geriatric Medicine, Keele University, April 1998*, at http: //www.roffe.freeserve.co.uk/keel.htm.

Roffe, D. and Roffe, C. 1995. 'Madness and care in the community: a medieval perspective', *British Medical Journal*, **311**, 1708-1712 [Accessed on the Internet 18 June 2003 at BMJ.com].

Rosen, G. 1964. 'The mentally ill and the community in Western and Central Europe during the late Middle Ages and the Renaissance', *Journal of the History of Medicine*, **19**, 377-388.

Rubin, M. 1987. *Charity and Community in Medieval Cambridge*, London & New York: Cambridge University Press.

Siraisi, N. 1990. *Medieval and Early Renaissance Medicine: An Introduction to Knowledge and Practice*, Chicago: University of Chicago Press.

Sutherland, D.W. 1967. 'Peytevin v. La Lynde', *Law Quarterly Review*, **83**, 527-546.

TNA: PRO - The National Archives: Public Record Office in Kew, UK.

Thiher, A. 1999. *Revels in Madness: Insanity in Medicine and Literature*, Ann Arbor: University of Michigan Press.

Turner W.J. 2010a. 'Town and country: a comparison of the treatment of the mentally disabled in late Medieval English common law and chartered boroughs', in W.J. Turner (ed.), *Madness in Medieval Law and Custom*, 17-38. Leiden & Boston: Brill.

Turner, W. 2010b. 'Silent testimony: emotional displays and lapses in memory as indicators of mental instability in Medieval English investigations', in W.J. Turner (ed.), *Madness in Medieval Law and Custom*, 81-95. Leiden and Boston: Brill.

Turner, W.J. 2013a. *Care and Custody of the Mentally Ill, Incompetent, and Disabled in Medieval England*, Cursor Mundi series. Leiden: Brepols.

Turner, W.J. 2013b. 'Defining Mental Afflictions in Medieval English Administrative Records', in C.J. Rushton (ed.), *Disability and Medieval Law: History, Literature, Society*, 134-157. Newcastle upon Tyne: Cambridge Scholars Publishing.

Waugh, S.L. 1988. *The Lordship of England: Royal Wardships and Marriages in English Society and Politics, 1217-1327*, Princeton: Princeton University Press.

Waugh, S.L. 1991. *England in the Reign of Edward III*, Cambridge Medieval Textbooks. Cambridge: Cambridge University Press.

Chapter 6
Disabling Masculinity: Manhood and Infertility in the High Middle Ages

Rachel Middlemass and Theresa Tyers

During the past few decades, women's experiences of infertility and its treatments have been explored by scholars from a range of academic disciplines, and there is now a very large body of work relating to these subjects.[1] More recently, interest in female fertility has extended to studies of men's experiences of infertility and sexual dysfunction, being particularly pronounced in social scientific disciplines and within the growing field of research into men's health.[2] Some working within these domains have suggested important links between male reproductive function and men's perceptions and construction of gendered identities, a suggestion predicated largely on the widely-accepted notion of sexual behaviour as key to defining gender roles.[3] Against a backdrop of growth in gender studies broadly and men's studies particularly, as well as in the health and medical humanities, research into the intersection of infertility and male identity has flourished,[4] although there remains an obvious asymmetry in the number of studies relating to women and men.

In response both to these sorts of studies and to a generally increased interest in the sexual and gendered identities of the past, several notable historical explorations of sexual dysfunction broadly, and impotence or infertility specifically, have also been produced.[5] But whilst the relationship between sexual and reproductive function and medieval masculine identity is introduced in several useful chapters and articles,[6] there is not yet to the best of our knowledge any extensive study devoted to these issues. This gap in the literature relating to medieval conceptions of male infertility and its repercussions for masculine identity seems incongruent with the existence of a considerable canon of research into other aspects of medieval sexual and gendered identities, a growing catalogue of work on medieval disability, and the availability of a sizeable corpus of medieval medical texts relevant to both these themes. In this paper we hope to contribute to redressing that gap by presenting an overview of some aspects of the relationship between sexual potency and manhood during the High Middle Ages.

We will begin by summarising some of the ways in which sexual dysfunction is and was understood by contemporary and medieval theorists.[7] We will then evaluate how restricted reproductive abilities interacted with dominant medieval cultural ideas and ideals for men's behaviour, particularly in terms of the significance of potency and fertility to particular 'types' of men's ability to fulfil social roles pertaining to marriage and fatherhood. On the basis of this analysis, we hope to evaluate whether or not infertility can be said to have been 'disabling' to men's efforts to achieve masculine status in medieval European society.

Infertility as Disability: Attitudes to Sexual Impairment in the Modern and Pre-Modern West

Any form of sexual dysfunction tends now to be fairly straightforwardly referred to as either a temporary or chronic 'impairment'. The issue of whether or not this impairment presents a legitimate disability is more complex: according to the World Health Organization's criteria the 'disabling' effects of an impairment depend upon its prevention or limitation of the performance of activities within or in the manner considered 'normal' for any human being.[8] Opinion is often divided in contemporary theory as to whether or not infertility and impotence should be defined in this way. Western medical organizations are usually reluctant to theorize infertility as disabling, in part because the activity that it restricts - that is, parenthood - is understood as something which is 'normal' in social rather than physiological terms. Infertility is further associated with the restriction of an ability which is, in any case, contingent on interaction with another person; in the event that this interaction never occurs the impairment need never be realized. Even supposing it is conceptually possible for an individual to be infertile by themselves, moreover, the impairment could in this case impose no possible restrictions on their usual range of activities and so would not meet the World Health Organisation's criteria for disability. The fact that infertility and impotence are not always chronic, may occur only in the union of one individual with a specific

[1] Slade 1981; Miall 1985; Kipper and Zadik 1996; Oddens, der Tonkelaar and Nieuwenhuyse 1999; Ulrich and Weatherall 2000; McQuillan et al 2004.
[2] Sabo and Gordon 1995; Browner and Sargent 1996; Lorber and Moore 1997; Drennan 1998; Doyal 2000.
[3] Dudgeon and Inhorn 2009, 8.
[4] Nachtigall, Becker and Wozny 1992; Mason 1993; Carmeli and Birenbaum-Carmeli 1994; Sabo and Gordon 1995; Webb and Daniluck 1999; Courtenay 2000; Inhorn, 2002, 2003; Gannon, Glover and Abel 2004; Dudgeon and Inhorn 2009.
[5] Brundage 1982; Morice et al 1995; Rider 2006; McLaren 2007.
[6] Murray 1990; Cadden 1993, 228-58; Bullough, 1994; Cooper and Leyser 2000; McLaren 2007, 25-49; van Eickels 2009.

[7] It should be noted that although the title of this paper refers only to infertility we will in fact also discuss impotence, or erectile dysfunction as it is now more usually termed. Infertility is usually agreed to denote the inability of a couple to conceive after at least one year of appropriately-timed and unprotected sexual intercourse. The sexual limitations associated with 'impotence', however, are myriad, often being distinguished as several different sorts of dysfunction relating to the several phases of a male sexual response cycle. Yakubu, Akanji and Oladiji summarise these as: disorders of desire; erectile dysfunction, disorders of ejaculation; disorders of orgasm; and failure of detumescence (Yakubu, Akanji and Oladiji 2007).
[8] Guimón 2001, 4.

other or others, and do not pose any serious threat in and of themselves to physical health, may also be cited as factors mitigating their 'disabling' effects.[9]

Pre-modern Western societies, however, evince a theoretical response to infertility which is consistent in recognizing its impact upon individuals' access to 'normal' social roles as disabling. Thus Jeremy Schipper argues that 'biblical, comparative ancient Near Eastern, and early rabbinic material all contain examples of infertility treated as a disability or illness',[10] examples whose equivalents may also be found in medieval European sources. Certainly, fertility represented a significant concern throughout the Middle Ages. Almost all medieval medical texts devoted some space to its consideration, and many explored it in detail, whilst instructions for diagnosing and treating reproductive disorders appear in most recipe collections.[11] The translation of older Arabic and ancient Greek medical texts into Latin during the 11th and 12th centuries no doubt catalyzed the surge of Western interest in these topics during that period. From the early 13th century, moreover, theoretical and medical texts began to be made available in vernacular languages, bringing medical knowledge to a wider audience of merchants, gentry and other educated laymen, as well as scholastics and university-trained physicians. Some of these texts related particularly to reproductive disorders,[12] and most contained practical as well as theoretical information to alleviate these. Detailed passages dealing with such subjects as diet and exercise were clearly intended not just to further readers' theoretical understanding of fertility, but to facilitate their diagnosis and treatment of a range of problems relating to it. Most vernacular texts assimilated treatments intended specifically for women and men within sections dealing with coitus and conception, an arrangement which contrasted with Greek and Roman authors' tendency to address male and female reproductive health separately. This newly integrative perspective on reproduction was perhaps a function of the frequent influence upon vernacular texts of Islamic and Byzantine medical encyclopaedias wherein, as Monica Green has demonstrated, female gynaecological and reproductive problems also tended to be discussed alongside treatments for male genital disorders.[13]

Despite this deep and widespread concern with reproductive health however, medieval theorists usually agreed with modern medics that sterility was not an absolute condition and that in most cases it could be treated and probably cured, albeit by recourse to what would today be judged

unusual means. One popular remedy which appears in several texts, including Constantinus Africanus' *De Coitu* and the *Practica Brevis* attributed to Platearius[14] called for ants and their eggs to be applied in a concoction to the testicles.[15] Alongside the same recipe in the Latin version of the c.1300 Anglo-Irish manuscript MS British Library Additional 15236 is a note specifying that it should be used only by those who were not totally impotent [*non sit totaliter impotens*],[16] testifying to the author's awareness of the complexity of the disorder. That impotence might be reversible is also acknowledged by the author of the *Practica Brevis*. Here, the causal explanations for impediments to conception [*impedimento conceptionis*] are followed by a lengthy discussion of the treatments appropriate to both men and women experiencing reproductive difficulties. Reiterating his point that most reproductive disorders could be treated, the writer concludes that only 'the defect which comes from the penis which is crooked or short is indeed incurable' [*Mes le vice qui vient del vit qui est tort ou cort si est incurable*].[17]

Neither ancient nor medieval theorists had any term corresponding precisely to 'disability' as it is now understood, but an examination of Greek and Latin semiotics reveals 'an awareness of a *de facto* social group whose numbers arouse unease or revulsion and connote a lesser state',[18] and who are described using certain words which correlate more or less precisely with 'disability'. The Greek words *adunatos*, *asthenés*, *akikus* and *anaperos* and the Latin terms *dehabilitus* and *infirmus*, for example, all imply 'physical or mental weakness, feebleness, the inability to function; the lack of performance; weakness in the mind or moral character; and social conditions such as poverty'.[19] Significantly, many of these terms suggest a deficit which is manifested and experienced in ways combining physiological with psychological and social facets. Contemporary theory, by comparison, clearly differentiates between these facets in its reference to two distinct models of disability. In the social model, disability is understood in exclusively social and political, rather than physical terms; in the medical model it is constructed as a straightforward physiological deficit or pathology requiring correction or cure. Edward Wheatley has recently claimed that 'the medical model of disability obviously does not apply to the Middle Ages, when medicine had hardly begun to develop into the institution that it is now'.[20] But whilst medicine may not have wielded the same institutional or discursive clout during the Middle Ages, many medieval theorists did treat sexual dysfunction as a physical defect and invested considerable intellectual effort in seeking and describing cures for it. As such, we would argue that medieval medical theorists in fact generally understood infertility as 'disabling' in *both*

---

[9] Although they deny that infertility directly threatens physical health, many clinicians and medical theorists do recognise that sexual dysfunction in any form can impose a heavy psychological burden, inducing 'depression, anxiety and debilitating feelings of inadequacy', and being closely (if not causally) related to such serious physical problems as heart disease, diabetes and obesity (Yakubu, Akanji and Oladiji, 50).
[10] Schipper 2007, 105.
[11] Cadden 1993, 229.
[12] For example, the collection of texts now in MS Cambridge Trinity College MS O.1.20.
[13] Green 1985, 83.

[14] Hunt 1994.
[15] Delany 1969.
[16] Hunt 1990, 240, fol.51 v.
[17] Hunt 1994, 245; fol.189v.
[18] Vlahogiannis 1998, 17.
[19] Vlahogiannis 1998, 17-18.
[20] Wheatley 2010, 9.

medical and social terms, often envisaging a complex and nuanced interrelationship between its physiological and social effects.

As well as their semiotic tendency to conflate social and physiological facets of disability, medieval scholars sometimes demonstrate confusion about - or perhaps simply disinterest in - the distinction between infertility and impotence as causes of male reproductive failure. In this they echo the attitudes of many classical scientific and medical writers, from whose work much of the corresponding medieval knowledge was derived, and who frequently collapsed the distinctions between infertility and impotence in generic descriptions of 'sterility'. Evidencing this tendency, (Pseudo-) Plutarch reported that:

> Diocles [says] that men are infertile either because some of them do not emit seed at all, or less than is required, or because the seed is infertile, or on account of a paralysis of the relevant parts, or on account of an obliquity of the penis, so that it cannot project the seed in a straight course, or because of the disproportion of the relevant parts with regard to the distance of the uterus.[21]

This conflation of infertility with other physiological forms of sexual dysfunction is similarly evident in practical texts such as the *Practica Brevis*, and the *De Coitu*. In part, the lack of interest in distinguishing between different forms of dysfunction reflects the fact that male fertility was often imagined in complex terms which did not allow for its reduction to genital function alone, even when the only visible sign of reproductive incapacity was an inability to achieve or sustain an erection. Thus, whilst women's fertility was usually linked unambiguously with the role of the uterus, men's reproductive capacity was understood as multi-faceted, with generative success being contingent upon the harmonious functioning of several other organs besides the genitals. Accordingly, fertility manuals of the high and later-middle ages linked male reproductive capacity primarily to the generative properties of men's brains, hearts and livers, and sometimes their kidneys, rather than their sexual organs.[22]

Even in these more complex conceptions of it, though, men's fertility was still ultimately defined in terms of their ability to generate semen and engage in sexual intercourse, factors which were, throughout the Middle Ages, linked more or less explicitly with humoural theory. Like most disorders, and whatever its underlying causes, 'sterility' was believed by many medieval physicians to arise principally from an imbalance in individuals' humoural complexion, particularly in heat, moisture, or both.[23] The

need to distinguish between specific forms of reproductive dysfunction was therefore further lessened by their supposedly shared origins in complexional imbalance. Writing in the late 11th century, Constantinus Africanus described the importance of humoural balance in ensuring male fertility:

> We will first discuss those men who are strong and excel in producing semen. Their testicles are of course hot and moist in the right proportion... Warmth increases desire and masculinity, whereas cold reduces desire and renders effeminate. If a man has warm testicles, therefore, he will be very lecherous and will conceive more boys; his pubic hair will appear at the right time, and also the hair on the rest of his body. But men with cold testicles will be effeminate and without desire; their hair will appear late and will be scanty around the pubis and groin. If the testicles are dry the man will have little desire and his semen will be scanty and weak. If they are moist, much semen will be produced and the hair will be flat and soft.[24]

The 13th-century physician Albertus Magnus likewise explained how male sterility could arise from a failure of the body to mature properly, a deficit to which he also attributed humoural origins. 'There are some men', he wrote, 'to whom semen does not come, because of a coldness and dryness of complexion.' [*Et quidam sunt quibus ex frigiditate et siccitate complexionis*].[25] Whilst Constantinus Africanus and Albertus Magnus appear to be describing infertility, the *Practica Brevis* author imagined other forms of sexual dysfunction - including impotence - as similarly underpinned by humoural imbalance. In a treatise on what he termed 'approximeron', he described 'an illness [whereby] when a man has started to have sexual intercourse and cannot accomplish it',[26] a condition which he attributed wholly to humoural origins.

The widespread acceptance of humoural causes for reproductive disorders is further attested to by the number of proposed remedies involving treatments to warm and thicken the blood, the medium that fostered procreation.[27]

closely linked to notions of its supernatural origins; appeals made via fasting, penance, exorcism and the invocation of saints were commonly advised as responses to magically-induced infertility or impotence. For more on this, and on the 'religious model' of disability, see Brundage 1982 and Wheatley 2010.

[24] Lindgren 2005, 5. *Dicemus in primis de illis hominibus qui fortes sont et prevalentes ad emittendum semen. Hiis nimirum testiculi sunt calidi et humidi temperate, verbi gracia... Calor enim auget appetitum velet masculinum, frigiditas autem diminuit appetitum et femininum reddit. Si ergo natura testium fuerit calida, multus erit appetitus luxurie et plures gignuntur masculine et tempestive oriuntur pili circa pectinem et circa reliquum corpus. Si vero fuerit frigida, effeminati erunt homines et appetites deest et pili oriuntur tarde et pauci circa ilia. Si vero fuerit sicca, modicus erit appetitus et modicum et debile semen. Quod si fuerit humida, semen redditur multum et pili oriuntur plani et molles* (Montero Cartelle 1983, 96-98).

[25] Cadden 1993, 147.

[26] MS Cambridge Trinity College 0.2.10, f.180v.

[27] Klein 1998, 31.

[21] van der Eijk 2000, 88. The Greek text is reproduced on p.87 of the same volume.

[22] Lindgren 2005, 5.

[23] Sexual dysfunction was also commonly attributed to witchcraft and other supernatural causes which are not discussed here. For a thorough treatment of the magical origins of infertility and impotence see Rider 2006. Perceptions of disability as a religious phenomenon are often

Many of the remedies in Anglo-Norman included among treatments in a copy of the *Practica Brevis* reiterate the necessity and feasibility of treating sterility in accordance with humoural theory. Thus the author calls for the use of 'warming' spices such as long pepper, cardamom, cloves and nutmeg. Some of these treatments echo those previously recommended by Constantinus Africanus, who also suggested the use of long pepper as a warming treatment to correct humoural imbalance, but who added that this should be taken in combination with horse beans to further increase the balancing effects.[28]

Against the backdrop of humoural theory the physiological and what we might describe as psychological causes of sexual dysfunction were, in some senses, both reduced to the level of the corporeal. Accordingly, Kenneth Boccafola suggests that the male condition known as *frigiditas* - a state which would now be understood as psychogenic - was seen as an organic defect, being 'universally understood as something natural, something pertaining to the personal physical constitution of the individual'.[29] On the other hand, classical and medieval theorists often acknowledged a whole range of impediments to intercourse or fertility which went beyond physiological defects. Aristotle, for example, cited variations in climate as a possible cause of infertility,[30] a notion which remained popular during the High and later Middle Ages. Specifically psychological causes might also be cited: the complex formulations of intercourse studied by Lindgren and others, in which the brain was supposed to play a vital part in generation, clearly suggested the contingency of successful reproduction on internal as well as external forces. Both Andreas Capellanus and Albertus Magnus described fantasy as an important component in achieving intercourse, the latter explaining that 'the mental picture of the opposite sex, imagined in the mind of a lover, is an important prerequisite to human mating because the image of a loveable woman has an exciting effect on a man'.[31] Indeed, in his commentary on Aristotle's *De animalibus* Albertus Magnus declared that the roots of sterility ultimately lay entirely in the soul rather than the body, even if they were manifested corporally.[32] John of Gaddesden offered similar advice in his early 14th century *Rosa Anglica*, urging men to sing bawdy songs, discuss sex openly, strike up conversations with beautiful women, and even observe intercourse in animals or other humans.[33] Gaddesden emphasised that erotic fantasy was especially important to men who were shy or impotent, reaffirming his awareness that sexual incapacity might have psychogenic as well as physiological or environmental causes. Sterility, moreover, was rarely considered in the neutral isolation of a purely medical context. Instead, it was almost always addressed within the broader context of generation and parenthoods, the social purposes or products of coitus. As such, the emphasis was on the need

to facilitate conception, rather than sex, and the pathology of sexual dysfunction was understood less as a simple, individual physiological deficit than as a fundamentally social problem pertaining to a couple's inability to procreate. The easy overlaps imagined in medieval theory between internal and external, psyche and soma, personal and social, thus maintained sexual dysfunction as a social, as well as a medical problem.

Although medieval theorists also conceived of sexual dysfunction as a medical problem to be corrected or cured, many discussions of medieval infertility did tend to focus on these social effects of reproductive impairment rather than on the impairment itself. In this, they have much in common with the social models of disability described by modern theorists, in which physiological impairments are considered principally in terms of their limitations on social role performance, rather than on physical capacity alone.[34] Since it prioritises social role over physical capacity, the social conception of disability challenges the argument that an inability to become a parent is objectively disabling because it is 'only' socially constructed as normal. The fact that relatively few adults live in complete sexual isolation, such that they have no opportunity to become parents, and that a majority of the world's adult population achieves parenthood, are also cited by those who support its recognition as a 'normal' human activity and the correspondingly 'disabling' limitations presented by chronic sexual dysfunction. It is useful here to bring in the additional term 'handicap' to refer specifically to these social components of impairment and disability - that is, to the manner and degree that the primary impairment and functional disability limit the performance of social roles.[35] To produce a handicap in the proper sense of the word, these disadvantages must pertain to social roles which are normal for an individual, both in relation to their age, gender, social status and so on, and in the light of any aspirations and life goals which they might have.[36] This latter point is particularly important in the context of masculinity, since gender identity is so closely linked with individuals' ability to conform to the socially constructed behavioural models which constitute gender norm. Any form of sexual dysfunction may have a direct negative impact upon sexual identity - itself a component of gender identity - but it may also affect gender identity less directly by inhibiting individuals' abilities to fulfil important aspects of their socially prescribed gender roles. The particular aspect of medieval (and indeed modern) men's gender role most clearly threatened by infertility and impotence is fatherhood, but sexual dysfunction also called into question men's ability to marry in medieval society. Since marriage and fatherhood were widely understood as the cornerstones of many forms of adult manhood, an inability to fulfil these roles might reasonably be expected to 'handicap' medieval masculinity. However, the extent to

---

[28] Delany 1969.
[29] Boccafola 1975, 47.
[30] Biller 2000, 258.
[31] Solomon 1997, 52.
[32] Resnick and Kitchell 2008, 509.
[33] Gaddesden 1516.

[34] Wiersma, DeJong and Orme 1988.
[35] Susser and Watson 1971.
[36] Guimón 2001, 4.

which this was in fact the case was, as we shall see, subject to significant variation.

Sexual Dysfunction and Social Roles: Some Impacts on 'Manly' Behaviour

Marriage

From the later 12th century, theoretical discussions of sexual dysfunction were increasingly focused on the legal ramifications of infertility and impotence. In late antique and early medieval societies, infertility had been little contested as a legitimate barrier to marriage. Indeed, sterility was cited in the first instance of divorce under ancient Roman tradition in 235 BC, when Carvilius Riga divorced his wife for her barrenness,[37] and Mesopotamian law permitted husbands either to divorce their wives or to take a second wife or handmaid if the first could not bear them no children.[38] Sterility was recognised as a condition which affected men too and was also grounds for women to bring a case for divorce. In the 6th century AD, Justinian added impotence to the list of legitimate reasons for divorcing under Roman law, stating that a woman or her parents could repudiate her husband if he had still proved unable to have sex with her after two years of marriage.[39]

During the 8th and 9th centuries, though, the question of fertility as grounds for divorce was reappraised. New distinctions were introduced relating to issues such as whether or not sterility had been a problem throughout the entire duration of a relationship or had developed after the relationship began.[40] Although women could sometimes still obtain annulments on the basis of their husbands' infertility, this became more difficult. In part, this change reflected an increasing emphasis among medical practitioners on the idea that infertility might be either 'naturally' temporary or able to be cured: for it to be accepted as a legitimate impediment to marriage, it had to be proven to be a permanent impairment. The legitimacy of infertility as a barrier to marriage was also affected by new challenges to the assumption that the principal (if not sole) purpose of marriage was procreation. The Gregorian reforms promoted an increased emphasis on chastity, even within marriage, so that a couple's failure to produce offspring might not be problematic so long as both parties freely chose to uphold chastity in their relationship. The negative impact of either party's infertility might then be mitigated to some extent by the fact that the range of 'normal' marital behaviours was extended to include chastity, with the range of normal or aspirational male behaviours concurrently extended to embrace non-procreative marital relations. In theory at least, therefore, infertile men need not be disabled in their roles and responsibilities as husbands, as long as both they and their spouse chose to uphold a chaste marriage.

If the production of children was no longer considered essential to fulfilling marital roles, though, the act of consummation was. An inability to have intercourse had been recognized as posing a challenge to marriage as early as the 8th century, and this was gradually developed into a comprehensive set of canon rules relating to impotence as an impediment.[41] Frankish and Anglo-Saxon penitentials had permitted women to divorce on the grounds of their husbands' impotence, even though they hadn't recognised infertility as a justification for so doing.[42] By the 13th century, theorists including Thomas Aquinas felt able to state explicitly that it was the act of penetration, rather than the possibility of conception, which was essential to the validation a marriage.[43] On the other hand, as with infertility, ecclesiastical courts tended increasingly to demand incontrovertible evidence of the permanent nature of husbands' impotence before they were willing to grant an annulment or divorce.[44] Accordingly it was, by 1215, a requirement of those seeking an annulment on the basis of impotence that they provide medical evidence attesting to the fact that their husband's sexual dysfunction related to a permanent physical defect. In his influential early 13th century tract *Summa confessorum*, which was widely disseminated across Europe, Thomas Chobham recommended that where impotence was alleged, 'wise matrons' [*sagaces matron*] be chosen 'to swear to inspect the genital members'. The women's report should then be used to support a judgement as to whether the subject 'has members suitable for intercourse or he has not'.[45]

To some extent, the implications of infertility and impotence for men's ability to marry were theoretically alleviated from the 12th or 13th century onwards, when it began to be recognised that these impairments were not necessarily perpetual. Meanwhile, the extension of chastity as an ideal for lay as well as religious men and women allowed infertile couples access to a legitimate - if little used - alternative to procreative marriage. There was, though, no equivalent safe haven for couples unable even to consummate their marriage, and for those men who suffered it, impotence remained a significant barrier to their ability to fulfil their socially prescribed roles as husbands. Male impotence could and did result in some wives' desertion of them.[46] Even after it had been recognised that some women were also physically incapable of coitus, moreover, impotence continued to be seen primarily as a defect in the male.[47] This was in contrast to infertility, for which women continued, in the main, to bear the burden of responsibility. Texts dealing with infertility did, admittedly, commonly include descriptions of tests intended to determine which partner was sterile; in his *De secretis mulierum* Psuedo Albertus Magnus referred to an older and apparently widely-known test involving adding bran of wheat to urine samples from

---

[37] Johnson, Coleman-Norton and Bourne 2003, 5.
[38] Bertman 2003, 277.
[39] Reynolds 1994, 16.
[40] Baumgarten 2004, 32.
[41] Murray 1990, 235.
[42] Örsy 1986, 23-4.
[43] McLaren 2007, 33.
[44] Boccafola 1975, 13-38.
[45] Murray 1990, 242-4.
[46] Butler 2006.
[47] Cadden 1993, 249; Bullough 1994, 41.

both parties. The mixture, Albertus advised, should be left for nine days and then re-inspected, whereupon 'if the defect is in the man, there will be worms in the pot; if the fault is the woman's, menses will be found in hers'.[48] The fault, however, was only relatively rarely found to be in the man, and there are many more examples of texts such as the *De conceptu*[49] which deal mostly with 'impediments to conception' arising from the female partner than those dealing with male infertility.[50]

Fatherhood

Impotence, rather than infertility, may then have posed the greater threat to men's ability to fulfil their roles as husbands. But either condition, if chronic, threatened to restrict or deny them access to fatherhood. The sense of infertility as disabling to the fulfilment of social roles has generally been considered by contemporary theorists almost exclusively in relation to women, for whom it is seen to inhibit the socially central role as mothers.[51] Until recently, indeed, infertility has been understood as peculiarly and disproportionately distressing to women than to men, a response thought to be provoked by the fact that cultural norms continue to emphasise the vital importance of motherhood to female identity.[52] Here, again, there is some overlap with ancient and medieval models, which were similarly more likely to emphasis the debilitating effects of infertility upon woman than upon men. There is no known male equivalent of the 1317 case of Thomassie, daughter of William Blancvilain, who sought to divorce her husband Thomas on grounds of his impotence and whose representative told the court that she 'is a virgin, and wants to be a mother'.[53]

In part, the lack of information about men's feelings on the subjects of sexual relationships and parenthood is a function of the fact that these have only relatively recently begun to be explored by historians of the medieval period. Certainly, there is still disagreement as to which aspects of fatherhood were particularly important to the construction of masculine identities. Vern Bullough has emphasised men's demonstrable engagement with heterosexual sexual relationships, stating that: 'Male sexual performance was a major key to being male... it was important for a man to keep demonstrating his maleness... especially by sexual action'.[54] Angus McLaren agrees that 'in the Middle Ages virility was prized and only fully proven by

siring offspring'.[55] Focusing more on the social aspects of fatherhood and fulfilment of familial obligations to continue blood lines, however, Derek Neal argues that: 'In a world where marriage and fatherhood so importantly signified manhood, inability to marry and to produce lineal heirs may have been more sorely missed than sexual activity *per se*'.[56] And if the importance of sexual relationships to the construction and maintenance of masculine identities is still under-theorized, the relative significance of father-son relationships remains virtually untouched. Ruth Karras offers a rare - albeit brief - comment on this aspect of men's identities when she suggests that 'it was the fact of patrilineal reproduction, rather than the relationship with a son, that contributed to medieval manhood'.[57]

In fact, all these facets of fatherhood probably mattered to medieval men, but with some important variations according to factors such as their age, social status and, of course, vocation. The most obvious difference perhaps relates to the importance of marriage and heterosexual sex to lay masculinities, as opposed to monastic men's purely symbolic marriage to the Church and subsequent avoidance of sexual relations. In this context, the potentially disabling effects of infertility and impotence posed a far greater threat to the maintenance of secular rather than religious masculinities. Indeed, there are some indications that a physical incapacity for sex - and even more particularly for sexual desire - could be positively advantageous to the attainment of masculine status in monastic circles. Ascetic theorists of masculinity based their vision of virility on the degree to which a man had transcended the desires of his body, so that the better able he was to resist sexual temptation the more 'manly' he became.[58] Rather than raising their masculine status, sexual desire threatened to undo it, reducing them to the level of secular men and women, upon whose all-consuming libidos and inability to control their own bodily fluxes many monastic writers poured scorn. In the late 12th century a young Hugh of Lincoln was rewarded with castration by a saint as a means of freeing him from his struggles with the flesh.[59] Somewhat less dramatically, his 13th century successor, Robert Grosseteste, expressed gratitude for his depressed libido, a condition which he attributed to a cooler humoural complexion than other men. To Grosseteste, this lack of libido was a blessing which freed him from the relentless sexual desires of other men, giving him an edge in the battle for monastic masculine status.[60]

Mitigating Infertility

These types of very different behavioural ideals were obviously important in determining the extent to which infertility and other sexual dysfunctions 'disabled', or indeed improved, men's access to masculine status. But

---

[48] Lemay 1981, 200-201.
[49] The text is of uncertain authorship and date: extant copies are attributed variously to Arnau de Villanova (1240-1311); Jean Jacme (d.1384) and Pierre Nadille (fl. 1369-74), personal physician to Charles II, king of Navarre.
[50] Conde Parrado, Montero Cartelle and Herrero Ingelmo 1999.
[51] Miall 1985.
[52] See for example Freeman, Boxer, Rickels, Tureck and Mastroianni 1985; Matthews and Matthews 1986; Nock 1987; Brand 1989; Ulbrich, Coyle and Llabre 1990; Wright *et al.*1991; Collins, Freeman, Boxer and Tureck 1992; Nachtigall, Becker and Wozny 1992; Jordan and Revenson 1999.
[53] Biller 2000, 20.
[54] Bullough 1994, 41.

[55] McLaren 2007, 38.
[56] Neal 2008, 121.
[57] Karras 2003, 166.
[58] Coon 2010, 9.
[59] *Ibid.*
[60] Murray 2008, 44.

other factors were also significant in mitigating men's inabilities - whether physical, psychogenic or vocational - to fulfil certain social roles. Of particular interest in the context of fertility are the several legitimate alternatives that medieval societies offered to biological fatherhood.

'Social Fathers': Alternatives to Biological Parenthood

'Social fatherhood' - the assumption of responsibility for parenting a child not biologically one's own - was fairly common in certain sections of Western medieval society. Monastic communities, for instance, whose members were (theoretically) disbarred from biological fatherhood, incorporated a range of quasi-parental and filial relationships were maintained. The most obviously paternal relationship was that between the abbot and his monks, and there is ample evidence in the writing of medieval abbots of a real sense of affection and responsibility for the brethren in their care. The 12th-century abbot Bernard of Clairvaux often addressed or referred to the monks at his own abbey as his 'sons' or 'children'. In a moving letter of c.1137 he writes during a long absence from Clairvaux: 'Unless I am mistaken this is the third time that my sons have been torn from me, weaned before their time. I am prevented from rearing the sons I have "begotten in the Gospel"'.[61] In a similar tone, Bernard praises Alvisus, Abbot of Anchin for his fatherly behaviour towards a previously troublesome monk at the time of that monk's death: 'Most appropriately', Bernard writes, 'you behaved as a father rather than a judge and tried, as a true father should, to satisfy the claims of charity and piety... At the first mention of your son's death your fatherly heart was touched'.[62]

Nor was social fatherhood the exclusive preserve of a religious life that theoretically excluded biological fatherhood. Secular men, too, might take on the role of 'social' father, whether or not they also had biological offspring or not. After the death of his biological father when he was eight, the tutor engaged for him by his mother provided Guibert of Nogent with a substitute father figure. Although he 'crushed' Guibert with the severity of the corporal punishments that he meted out, Guibert nevertheless wrote of his tutor that:

> In other ways he made it quite plain that he loved me as well as he did himself. With such watchful care did he devote himself to me, with such foresight did he secure my welfare against the spite of others and teach me on what authority I should beware of the dissolute manners of some who paid court to me, and so long did he argue with my mother about the elaborate richness of my dress, that he was thought to

guard me as a parent, not as a master, and not my body alone, but my soul as well. As for me, considering the dull sensibility of my age and littleness, I conceived much love for him in response, in spite of the many weals with which he furrowed my tender skin, so that not through fear, as is common in those of my age, but through a sort of love deeply implanted in my heart, I obeyed him in utter forgetfulness of his severity.[63]

Among gentry and merchant classes, the practice of sending apprentices out to learn their trade as small boys - often only eleven or twelve and sometimes even younger - allowed some men to fulfil a fatherly role in relation to them, particularly since these boys usually remained in their households for several years. Apprentices certainly stood in a position very similar to that of children in their households, and in fact many of them were related either more or less distantly to members of the family which took them in. Like children, they were expected to provide their masters with unquestioning obedience, as well as their physical labour, but in return they often received moral guidance and perhaps formal schooling, as well as the vocational training they were officially there to acquire.[64] In situations where apprentices were fairly closely related to their masters, or where their master had no children of their own to follow them into the trade, the quasi-parental nature of apprenticeship might well have assumed a close emotional tie too.[65]

Higher up the social scale, access to social fatherhood could be provided via traditions of wardship or 'fostering', whereby children were raised in the households of associates of their biological families in order to learn skills, manners, and expertise, or to make important social connections - including marriage - which would be advantageous to them in later life.[66] Even where children were raised within the households of their own biological families, the much fuller role of extended kin throughout the period meant that male relatives other than the father might well have access to quasi-parental relationships with children who were not their own. There is some evidence in stories such as *The Song of Roland*, for example, that maternal uncles, in particular, often played an important role in rearing their sisters' offspring, being described by Mary McLaughlin as 'male mothers' to them.[67]

[61] James 1953, 214. *Ecce hoc tertie, nisi fallor, avulsa sunt a me viscera mea. Parvuli ablactati sunt ante tempus: ipsos quos per Evangelium genui, non licit educare* (Mabillon 1839, 301).

[62] James 1953, 92. *Patrem quippe vos cognovistis, ut res exigebat, non judicem. Ideoque quod pietatis, quod charitatis est, ut vere filio pater impendere studuistis... Ad unum nempe nuntium de morte filii, paterna viscera commota sunt* (Mabillon 1839, 171).

[63] Benton 1984, 49. *Quamvis ergo tanta me severitate deprimeret, alias tamen omnibus modis propatulum faciebat, quod me pene non alia, quam se charitate diligeret. Adeo nempe vigili mihi solicitudine incumbebat, adeo propter quorundam invidentias saluti meae providebat, obsoletos aliquorum, qui mihi observabant, mores, quanta caverem auctoritate docebat, matrem super cultissimo mearum vestium apparatu tantisper urgebat, ut non paedagogi, sed parentis partem, non corporis mei tutelam, sed animae curam agree putaretur. Mihi vero, licet pro aetate hebeti atque pusiolo, tanta penes eum vicissitudo amoris incesserat, licet gratis multotiens cuticulam meam multis vibicibus persulcaret, ut non metu, qui in aequavis assolet, sed nescio quo medullitus insito amore, ei totius ejus asperitatis oblitus, obsequerer* (Labande 1981, 36-8).

[64] Singman 1999, 26.

[65] Epstein 1991, 105-6.

[66] Kuefler 2003.

[67] McLaughlin 1974, 178.

Conclusions

Medieval European society provided several legitimate alternatives to biological fatherhood. Access to these alternative forms of parenting, as well as the existence of some masculine behavioural models within which biological fatherhood played no part at all, theoretically mitigated the 'disabling' effects of infertility for at least some of the men affected by it. For men whose social standing demanded celibacy, valourized virginity, and demonized sexual desire, dysfunctions in libido or sexual performance might actually be helpful in the attainment of masculine status, and certainly ought not to have been disabling. The quasi-parental social roles available to (at least some) men within religious communities may have helped ease tensions arising from their theoretical disbarment from biological fatherhood.

But whilst access to social fatherhood perhaps addressed some of these tensions, the extent to which it truly mitigated the effects of generative limitations either for religious or, certainly, for lay men, depends on variations in the ways in which fatherhood was conceptualized and valued within different constructions of manhood. If, in the context of fatherhood, masculine status was conferred chiefly by the act of parenting, with the myriad responsibilities and tests of self-restraint entailed by that, then access to social fatherhood clearly could mitigate the 'disabling' effects of chronic infertility or impotence on men's ability to fulfil a 'normal' social role. If, on the other hand, masculinity was equated principally with sexual potency alone, then access to social roles mimicking that of the father would not be sufficient to alleviate the threat posed by sexual dysfunction. Vern Bullough has been a vocal proponent of the latter interpretation, arguing that the medieval male was defined primarily 'in terms of sexual performance, measured, rather simply, as his ability to get an erection',[68] such that evidence of any lack of virility necessarily threatened male identity. Infertility, as well as impotence, is also often explicitly linked with notions of dominant manhood: Marcia Inhorn writes that, 'the "failure" of sperm to impregnate poses one of the greatest challenges to hegemonic masculinity'.[69] There is here some suggestion that, even if parenting is not understood as central to the gendered identities of individual men, the masculine mandate nevertheless emphasises the ability to reproduce.

Speaking in broader terms about the interaction of disability and gender, Jenny Morris argues that 'the social definition of masculinity is inextricably bound up with a celebration of strength, or perfect bodies. At the same time, to be masculine is not to be vulnerable'.[70] This close association between masculinity and physical perfection, completeness, and strength is certainly reflected in the work of many medieval theorists. Their common emphasis on the male's perfect and intact physicality presumably made any form of physical weakness or defect, whether arising from disability or disease, a serious threat to men's capacity to meet the most highly prized masculine ideals.

In order to present an overview of some of the challenges presented by sexual dysfunction to specifically masculine identities, this paper has considered sexual dysfunction primarily as it affected men alone. In reality, though, the disabling effects of infertility or impotence on individuals' ability to fulfil their socially prescribed roles relate at least as much to how these impairments affected men and women together. This certainly seems to have been medieval theorists' understanding of the situation; impotence and infertility were increasingly imagined by them as a problem for the couple, and perhaps even for the community, rather than for the individual. Medical writers were ever more accepting of the idea that any form of sexual or reproductive dysfunction might result from deficiencies in either partner or from the specific combination of partners. In the contemporary social model of disability, the effects of impairment on social role rarely relate to the roles of either sex in isolation from the other. The social roles of men and women are inextricably interlinked, so that that the effects of any impairment on the ability of one sex to fulfil the roles ascribed to it is likely also to affect the other. Thus, for example, although medieval societies upheld some masculine behavioural models which did not include biological fatherhood, and although they provided legitimate alternatives for men in the form of social fatherhood roles, women's behavioural ideals were (and are still) very closely associated with the role of mother. As such, a husband's infertility or impotence impinged not only on his own ability to fulfil his social role, but on that of his spouse as well. This wider impact of men's procreative limitations may help to explain why, despite the existence of a broad range of theoretical alleviations of its effects, men's sexual dysfunction seems to have remained widely stigmatized throughout the Middle Ages and beyond.

---

[68] Bullough 1994, 43.
[69] Inhorn et al 2009, 4-5.

[70] Morris 1997, 22.

Bibliography

Baumgarten, E. 2004. *Mothers and Children: Jewish Family Life in Medieval Europe.* New Jersey: Princeton University Press.

Benton, J.F. (ed.) 1984. *Self and Society in Medieval France: The Memoirs of Guibert of Nogent.* Toronto: University of Toronto Press.

Bertman, S. 2003. *Handbook to Life in Ancient Mesopotamia.* Oxford and New York: Oxford University Press.

Biller, P. 2000. *The Measure of Multitude: Population in Medieval Thought.* Oxford and New York: Oxford University Press.

Boccafola, K. 1975. *The Requirement of Perpetuity for the Impediment of Impotence.* Rome.

Brand, H.J. 1989. 'The influence of sex differences on the acceptance of infertility', *Journal of Reproductive and Infant Psychology* 7, 127-31.

Browner, C.H. and Sargent, C.F. 1996. 'Anthropology and studies of human reproduction', in C.F. Sargent and T.M. Johnson (eds), *Medical Anthropology: Contemporary Theory and Method (2nd edition)*, 219-34. Westport: Praeger.

Brundage, J.A. 1982. 'The problem of impotence', in J.A. Brundage and V. Bullough (eds), *Sexual Practices and the Medieval Church*, 135-40. Buffalo: Prometheus Books.

Bullough, V. 1994. 'On being a male in the Middle Ages', in C.A. Lees (ed.), *Medieval Masculinities: Regarding Men in the Middle Ages*, 31-45. Minnesota: University of Minnesota Press.

Caddon, J. 1993. *Meanings of Sex Difference in the Middle Ages.* Cambridge: Cambridge University Press.

Carmeli, Y.S. and Birenbaum-Carmeli, D. 1994. 'The predicament of masculinity: towards understanding the male's experience of infertility treatments', *Sex Roles* 30, 663-77.

Collins, A., Freeman, E.W., Boxer, A.S. and Tureck, R. 1992. 'Perceptions of infertility and treatment stress in females as compared with males entering in vitro fertilization treatment', *Fertility and Sterility* 57, 350-56.

Conde Parrado, P., Montero Cartelle, E., and Herrero Ingelmo, M.C (eds and trans (into Spanish)) 1999. *Tractatus de conceptu, Tractatus de sterilitate mulierum.* (Lingüítica y Filología, 37). Valladolid: Secretariado de Publicaciones e Intercambio Editorial, Universidad de Vallodolid.

Coon, L.L. 2010. *Dark Age Bodies: Gender and Monastic Practice in the Early Medieval West.* Pennsylvania: University of Pennsylvania Press.

Cooper, K. and Leyser, C. 2000. 'The gender of grace: impotence, servitude and manliness in the fifth-century West', *Gender and History* 12, 536-51.

Courtenay, W.H. 2000. 'Constructions of masculinity and their influence on men's well-being: a theory of gender and health', *Social Science and Medicine* 50, 1385-1401.

Delany, P 1969. 'Constantinus Africanus' *De Coitu*: a translation', *The Chaucer Review* 4, 55-65.

Doyal, L. 2000. 'Gender equality in health: debates and dilemmas', *Social Science and Medicine* 51, 931-39.

Drennan, M. 1998. 'Reproductive health: new perspectives on men's participation', *Population Reports Series J, Family Planning Programs* 46, 1-35.

Dudgeon, M.R. and Inhorn, M.C. 2009. 'Gender, masculinity, and reproduction: anthropological perspectives', in M.C. Inhorn (ed.), *Reconceiving the Second Sex: Men, Masculinity, and Reproduction*, 72-102. Oxford and New York: Berghahn Books.

van Eickels, K. 2009. 'Männliche Zeugungsunfähigkeit im mittelalterlichen Adel', *Medizin, Gesellschaft, und Geschichte. Jahrbuch des Instituts für Geschichte der Medizin der Robert Bosch Stiftung* 28, 73-95.

van der Eijk, P.J. (ed. and trans) 2000. *Diocles of Carystus: a Collection of the Fragments with Translation and Commentary.* 2 Volumes: Volume 1. Leiden: Brill.

Epstein, S.A. 1991. *Wage Labor and Guilds in Medieval Europe.* North Carolina: The University of North Carolina Press.

Freeman, E.W., Boxer, A.S., Rickels, K., Tureck, R. and Mastroianni, L. 1985. 'Psychological evaluation and support in a programme of in vitro fertilization and embryo transfer', *Fertility and Sterility* 43, 48-53.

Gaddesden, J. *Rosa anglica practica medicine.* Venice: Bonetus Locarellus.

Gannon, K., Glover, L. and Abel, P. 2004. 'Masculinity, infertility, stigma and media reports', *Social Science & Medicine* 59, 1169-75.

Green, M. 1985. *The Transmission of Ancinet Theories of Female Phusiology and Disease Through the Early Middle Ages.* PhD Dissertation, Princeton University.

Guimón, J. 2001. *Inequity and Madness: Psychosocial and Human Rights Issues.* New York: Springer.

Hunt, T. 1990. *Popular Medicine in Thirteenth-Century England.* Cambridge: D.S. Brewer.

Hunt, T. 1994. *Anglo-Norman Medicine: 1 Roger Frugard's* Chirurgia *and the* Practica Brevis *of Platearius.* Cambridge: D.S. Brewer.

Inhorn, M.C. 2002. 'Sexuality, masculinity, and infertility in Egypt: potent troubles in the marital and medical encounters', *Journal of Men's Studies* 10, 342-59.

Inhorn, M.C. 2003. '"The worms are weak": male infertility and patriarchal paradoxes in Egypt', *Men and Masculinities* 5, 236-56.

Inhorn, M.C., Tjørnhøj-Thomsen, T., Goldberg, H. and la Cour Mosegaard, M. 2009. 'Introduction', in M.C. Inhorn, T. Tjørnhøj-Thomsen, H. Goldberg, and M. la Cour Mosegaard (eds), *Reconceiving the Second Sex: Men, Masculinity, and Reproduction*, 1-20. Oxford and New York: Berghahn.

James, B.S. (ed and trans.) 1953. *The Letters of St. Bernard of Clairvaux.* London: AMS Press.

Johnson, A.C., Coleman-Norton, P.R., and Bourne, F.C. 2003. *Ancient Roman Statutes. A Translation with Introduction, Commentary, Glossary, and Index.* New Jersey: The Lawbook Exchange, Ltd.

Jordan, C. and Revenson, T.A. 1999. 'Gender differences in coping with infertility: a meta-analysis', *Journal of Behavioural Medicine* **22**, 341-58.

Karras, R. 2003. *From Boys to Men: Formations of Masculinity in Late Medieval Europe*. Pennsylvania: University of Pennsylvania Press.

Kipper, D.A. and Zadik, H. 1996. 'Functional infertility and femininity: a comparison of infertile women and their mothers', *Journal of Clinical Psychology* **53**, 375-82.

Klein, M. 1998. *A Time to be Born. Customs and Folklore of Jewish Birth*. Philadelphia: Jewish Publication Society.

Kuefler, M.S. 2003. 'Male friendship and the suspicion of sodomy in twelfth-century France', in S.A. Farmer and C.B. Pasternack (eds), *Gender and Difference in the Middle Ages*, 145-181. Minnesota: University of Minnesota Press.

Lemay, H.R. 1981. 'William of Saliceto on human sexuality', *Viator* **12**, 165-81.

Lindgren, A. 2005. *The Wandering Womb and the Peripheral Penis: Gender and the Fertile Body in Late Medieval Infertility Treatises (France)*. PhD Thesis. University of California.

Lorber, J. and Moore, L. 1997. *Gender and the Social Construction of Illness*. Thousand Oaks, CA: AltaMira Press.

Mabillon, D.J. 1839. *Sancti Bernardi Abbatis Clarae-Vallensis Opera Omnia* vol. I. Paris: Daume Fratres.

McLaughlin, M.M. 1974. 'Survivors and surrogates: children and parents from the ninth to the thirteenth centuries' in L. de Mause (ed.), *The History of Childhood*, 101-81. New York: Harper and Row.

McLaren, A. 2007. *Impotence: A Cultural History*. Chicago and London: University of Chicago Press.

McQuillan, J., Greil, A.L., White, L. and Jacob, M.C. 2004. 'Frustrated fertility: infertility and psychological distress among women', *Journal of Marriage and Family* **65(4)**, 1007-1018.

Mason, M.C. 1993. *Male Infertility: Men Talking*. New York: Routledge.

Matthews, R. and Matthews, A.M. 1986. 'Infertility and childlessness: the transition to non-parenthood', *Journal of Marriage and the Family* **48**, 641-49.

Miall, C.E. 1985. 'Perceptions of informal sanctioning and the stigma of involuntary childlessness', *Deviant Behaviour* **6**, 383-405.

Montero Cartelle, E. (ed. And trans. into Spanish) 1983. *Constantine the African: Liber de Coitu: El tratado de andrologia, estudio y edicion critica*. Santiago de Compostela: Universidad de Santiago de Compostela.

Morice, P, Josset, P., Chapron, C. and Dubuisson, J.B. 1995. 'History of Infertility', *Human Reproduction Update* **1**, 497-504.

Morris, J. 1997. 'A feminist perspective', in C. Davies and A. Pointon (eds), *Framed: Interrogating Disability in the Media*, 21-33. London: BFI Publishing.

Murray, J. 1990. 'On the origins and role of "wise women" in causes for annulment on the grounds of male impotence', *Journal of Medieval History* **16**, 235-49.

Murray, J. 2008. 'One flesh, two sexes, three genders?' in L.M. Bitel and F. Lifschitz (eds), *Gender and Christianity in Medieval Europe: New Perspectives*, 34-51. Pennsylvania: University of Pennsylvania Press.

Neal, D. 2008. *The Masculine Self in Late Medieval England*. Chicago: University of Chicago Press.

Nachtigall, R.D., Becker, G., and Wozny, M. 1992. 'The effects of gender-specific diagnosis on men's and women's response to infertility', *Fertility and Sterility* **57**, 113-21.

Nock, S.L. 1987. 'The symbolic meaning of childbearing', *Journal of Family Issues* **8**, 373-93.

Oddens, B.J., den Tonkelaar, I. and Nieuwenhuyse, H. 1999. 'Psychosocial experience in women facing fertility problems - a comparative survey', *Human Reproduction* **14**, 255-61.

Örsy, L.M. 1986. *Marriage in Canon Law: Texts and Comments, Reflections and Questions*. Delaware: Gracewing Publishing.

Resnick, I. M. and Kitchell, K. (trans) 2008. *Albert the Great's Questions Concerning Aristotle's 'On Animals'*. Fathers of the Church, Medieval Continuation 9. Washington DC: Catholic University of America Press.

Reynolds, P.L. 1994. *Marriage in the Western Church: The Christianization of Marriage During the Patristic and Early Medieval Periods*. Leiden: Brill Academic Publishers.

Rider, C. 2006. *Magic and Impotence in the Middle Ages*. Oxford: Oxford University Press.

Sabo, D. and Gordon, D.F. 1995. 'Rethinking men's health and illness: the relevance of gender studies', in D. Sabo and D.F. Gordon (eds), *Men's Health and Illness: Gender, Power, and the Body*, 1-21. London: Sage Publications.

Schipper, J. 2007. 'Disabling Israelite Leaderships: 2 Samuel 6:23 and other images of disability in the Deuteronomistic history', in H. Avalos, S.J. Melcher, and J. Schipper, (eds), *This Abled Body: Rethinking Disabilities in Biblical Studies*, 103-114. Atlanta: Society of Biblical Literature.

Singman, J.L. 1999. *Daily Life in Medieval Europe*. Westport: Greenwood Press.

Slade, P. 1981. 'Sexual attitudes and social role orientation in infertile women', *Journal of Psychosomatic Research* **25**, 183-6.

Susser, N.W. and Watson, W. 1971. *Sociology in Medicine* (2nd edition). London, Oxford: Oxford University Press.

Ulbich, P.M., Coyle, A.T. and Llabre, M.M. 1990. 'Involuntary childlessness and marital adjustment: his and hers', *Journal of Sex and Marital Therapy* **16**, 147-58.

Ulrich, M. and Weatherall, A. 2000. 'Motherhood and infertility: viewing motherhood through the lens of infertility', *Feminism and Psychology* **10**, 323-36.

Vlahogiannis, N. 1998. 'Disabling bodies', in D. Montserrat (ed.), *Changing Bodies, Changing Meanings: Studies on the Human Body in Antiquity*, 13-36. London: Routledge.

Webb, R. and Daniluck, J. 1999. 'The end of the line: infertile men's experience of being unable to produce a child', *Men and Masculinities* **2**, 6-25.

Wheatley, E. 2010. *Stumbling Blocks Before the Blind: Medieval Constructions of a Disability*. Michigan: University of Michigan Press.

Wiersma, D., DeJong, A. and Ormel. J. 1988. 'The Groningen Social Disabilities Schedule: development, relationship with I.C.I.D.H. and psychometric properties', *International Journal of Rehabilitation Research* **11**, 37-44.

Wright, J., Bissonnette, F., Duchesne, C., Benoit, J., Sabourin, S. and Girard, Y. 1991. 'Psychosocial distress and infertility: men and women respond differently', *Fertility and Sterility* **55**, 100-108.

Yakubu, M.T., Akanji M.A., and Oladiji, A.T. 2007. 'Male sexual dysfunction and methods used in assessing medicinal plants with aphrodisiac potentials', *Pharmacognosy Reviews* **1**. 49-56.

Chapter 7
Speechless: speech and hearing impairments as problem of medieval normative texts - theological, natural-philosophical, legal[1]

Irina Metzler

Introduction

In an illumination in a *Bible moralisée* of the 13th century,[2] old Zacharias is depicted struck dumb by the angel Gabriel and not able to speak until the day the prophesied birth of John the Baptist comes to pass. This illustrates the passage in Luke 1:18-20: 'and when Zacharias came out of the temple he could not speak to the people but beckoned to them and remained speechless'. In this chapter, I will be addressing the chronologically and geographically diverse attitudes to and status of (congenitally) deaf people during the western European Middle Ages, and especially those concomitant legal problems which, among the many different physical manifestations of impairment, elicited the most complex legal responses, namely the absence of language due to speech and hearing impairments. Most congenitally deaf people, in the days before special education became available, were also functionally mute, even if physically capable of speech, because to learn to speak one must first be able to hear spoken language, hence in the following argument both disabilities will be discussed together. 'Legal' will be understood in its widest context, hence not just medieval canon and civil law, but also other normative texts that shaped or reflected medieval mentalities. Thus theological texts and natural philosophy are just as relevant for my argument as codes of law. While after the beginning of the 14th century some medieval authorities began to realise that language acquisition is a social event, other authorities still regarded the deaf as equivalent to mentally impaired, which gives us an indication of precisely that diversity of medieval mentalities mentioned above.

Normative aspects of speech and hearing problems start at the beginning. 'In the beginning was the Word, and the Word was with God, and the Word was God'. This is in the familiar English of the King James version; the Latin of the Vulgate reads: *'In principio erat Verbum et Verbum erat apud Deum et Deus erat Verbum'* (John 1:1). The importance of the word, of verbal communication, of speech, is clear from the outset. The implication of the spoken word is that it has to have a listener, a hearer, Latin *auditor* - what then about people who cannot hear?

Biblical textual references set the scene for the medieval theological and cultural 'problem' of the deaf. There are actually very few references to deaf people in the Bible. In the oft-quoted passage in Leviticus 21 on proscriptions concerning the physically-impaired the deaf are absent. Blind, lame, crooked backed people and people with various other visible 'blemishes' are not permitted to make sacrifices at the altar, i.e. to become priests, but the deaf are not excluded. But then deafness does not have any visible signs, since in outward appearance the deaf person is in no way different from the hearing person. So if the prime concern in Leviticus was to exclude people who gave visible 'offence', then there was no reason to exclude the deaf.

About the only other Old Testament instance where the deaf are mentioned in a non-metaphoric context is also in Leviticus 19:14, in the simple exhortation 'Thou shalt not curse the deaf, nor put a stumbling block before the blind' (in the Latin of the Vulgate: *non maledices surdo nec coram caeco pones offendiculum*). In the New Testament we have one, and only one, of Christ's many healing miracles where he cures a man who had been congenitally deaf (Mark 7:32-7). The passage that really had influence over how deaf people were regarded in subsequent times, and which to an extent underpinned an ancient and medieval philosophical paradigm, was Paul's letter to the Romans: 'So then faith cometh by hearing, and hearing by the word of God. But I say, Have they not heard? (in the Latin of the Vulgate: *ergo fides ex auditu auditus autem per verbum Christi sed dico numquid non auditum*). The phrase *fides ex auditu*, which actually refers to people - the Jews in the immediate context of the passage - who are *willing* (or unwilling) to hear the apostolic message, had later been misinterpreted and misrepresented so that it came to signify people who are *able* (or unable) to hear. The implications are, according to Augustine, that the suffering of blind or deafmute children is even worse than that of their parents, because following the words of the apostle Paul it is impossible to acquire the faith if one is deaf.[3] If the deaf could not demonstrate satisfactorily that they had understood enough of the creed to be received into Christian communion, neither could they confess their sins since they could not hear the questions of a confessor. In theological terms, faith can only be acquired and understood through hearing the teachings of Christ, consequently in social and legal terms deafmutes, who cannot be educated intellectually, cannot occupy a full place in law and have to be excluded from religious practices - or so the grand narrative goes.

[1] This essay arose from a paper presented at the 4th Disease and Disability workshop held at the University of Nottingham in 2010. While Woolgar's (2006) eponymous book on the senses in late medieval England comprehensively covers *intact* sensory perception, disabled or *non-functional* senses are not covered in the same fashion, hence deafness merited only a cursory mention.
[2] Toledo, Chapter of the Cathedral, Bible moralisée, fol. 1v

[3] Werner 1932, 74; cf. Augustine, *Contra Julian. Pelagian.*, III, cap. 4, *Patrologiae Latinae* (ed. Migne), vol. 44, col. 707: *'Quod vitium etiam ipsam impedit fidem, Apostolo testante, qui dicit: Igitur fides ex auditu'*.

Definitions

Congenital deafness is the rarest form of deafness. In contemporary Britain only about two in every 1000 infants are born with a hearing impairment that affects both ears, and even then there are great variations ranging from partial hearing loss to profound deafness. Deafmuteness was often caused by congenital deafness alone, since a deaf person never learned to utter an intelligible sound because they could not hear such sounds in the first place. 'Mute' in this context means the inability to utter meaningful speech, not the inability to utter any sound whatsoever. Congenital deafness in children was often only noticed quite some time after birth, and generally noticed much later than total muteness. Congenital deafness would have gone pretty much unnoticed for the first few months of a baby's life, because babies interact with their carers on communication based on body language as much as speech. Because an infant's language development follows even later than the developmental stage of reacting to other people's speech, true congenital deafmutes were therefore only recognised when their deafness was noticed, not by their lack of speaking ability.

As most mute people were first and foremost congenitally deaf and had simply not been enabled to learn speech even though physically capable of it, they were in effect *functionally* mute: such people often appear in the Latin sources as *muti*. People who were only deaf, but retained the ability of speech, especially those who had acquired their deafness later in life, through age, illness or injury, were termed *surdi*. Both terms were nevertheless very fluid and used interchangeably if referring to congenital conditions.

However, people who had acquired deafness later in life quite obviously demonstrated that deafness and muteness were not invariably linked, since many who lost their hearing were able to continue speaking, even if perhaps their speech deteriorated over time.[4] If they had been literate before their impairment they will have been able to continue communication by reading and writing - such seems to have been the case of the Spanish nun Teresa de Cartagena in the mid-15th century, who had acquired deafness in her late teens or early twenties.[5] Teresa mentions in her writings that she has been deaf for 20 years, but before she lost her hearing she had attended the University of Salamanca, so that she will have been highly literate, which meant that after becoming impaired she was able to find solace in reading and meditating: 'I must recur to my books which have wondrous graftings from healthful groves'.[6]

How the loss of a sense affects a person is examined by Jean de Jandun, a French scholastic in the early 14th century, who in his questions *Super de sensu* compared a child growing up in total isolation to a person impaired by hearing and speech loss:

> It has been said that because such a mute has not heard any meaningful speech, he cannot utter any. The question is: if a boy were reared in a forest, where he had never heard any kind of language, whether he would speak any language ... Likewise there is no habit of any speech unless through the social intercourse of men, and hence I say that he would not speak a language; he could well from natural appetite form sounds, but no consistent expressions unless he were later to have intercourse with others.[7]

What is not just interesting as an intellectual observation, but downright revolutionary in terms of how the deaf were perceived, is Jean's statement that the acquisition of verbal language is not innate but a social event.

Another natural philosopher of the early 14th century, Marsilius of Inghen, also theorised the effects of a child growing up in isolation and compared the effects on language development to that of a mute. Marsilius also rejected the notion of Hebrew as the 'natural' language as a 'silly and ridiculous' idea. Furthermore he said 'that that boy would remain mute until he was established by other men in a definite language; but if there were two boys placed together ... these could mutually set up between themselves a new language'.[8] The novel idea Marsilius therefore introduced was that the desire for communication was innate to human beings, irrespective of their faculties or circumstances. Thus at the turn of the 13th to the 14th century it was recognised that communication relied on socialisation of the individual at an early stage in life.

Furthermore, Jean de Jandun had questioned the widely-accepted ancient idea that there was a sympathetic association between the nerves of the ear and the vocal organs, so that the deaf were incurably speechless as well. Explaining why congenitally deaf people are also speech impaired Jean said in contrast:

> that someone congenitally deaf is necessarily dumb because anyone who cannot learn how to form meaningful speech at will is in that way necessarily dumb. This is self-evident, because knowing how to form meaningful speech at will comes about only through habit and social intercourse with people, but someone congenitally deaf cannot become accustomed to the expression of meaningful speech, because this requires that he hears speech of this kind.[9]

---

[4] Rée 1999, 7.
[5] Seidenspinner-Núñez 1998, 9-11.
[6] *Ibid.*

[7] Crombie 1996, 276-7; Joannes de Janduno, *Quaestiones super Parvis naturalibus*, Venetiis, 1589, f. A7 recto.
[8] Crombie 1996, 277; Marsilius of Inghen, *Quaestiones de sensu et sensato*, q. 3, quodlibet 1, MS Erfurt F.334, fol. 7 (8) recto, translated following *Le 'Quaestiones De Sensu' attribute a Oresme e Alberto di Sassonia* [=Nicholas Oresme and Albert of Saxony], a cura di Jole Agrimi, Florence, 1983.
[9] Crombie 1996, 284; Joannes de Janduno, *Quaestiones super Parvis naturalibus*, 'Super de sensu', q. 7.

More importantly, ideas such as those of Jean and Marsilius of Inghen opened the way for systematic measures to be developed which enabled the hearing impaired to more fully participate in society, since their theories removed the association between congenital deafness and intellectual impairment. The prevailing notion had been that the congenitally deaf were also incapable of speech, which in turn meant they were incapable of rational thought, according to antique and medieval theories of cognition. Aristotle, for example, had said that of all the senses sight might be superior in gathering information, but hearing served a greater role in shaping intelligence, since it made possible rational discourse; he furthermore stated that congenitally blind people were more intelligent than congenitally deaf or mute people.[10] For the medieval period an example from the mid-12th century may suffice: in his *Cosmographia* Bernard Silvestris stated: 'If men had deaf ears, letters would perish'.[11]

Once congenital deafness was regarded as purely that, deafness alone, and not a mental impairment, attention could begin to focus on the problem of how the hearing could communicate with the non-hearing. It nevertheless took until the 17th century for Girolamo Cardano to insist that the deaf were just as intelligent as the rest of humanity and could be educated by visual methods.[12] During the Renaissance various authorities built upon the pioneering work of Jean de Jandun. One such figure was Marin Mersenne, writing on language and music in the 1620s and 1630s. For the benefit of deaf people he drew up a table showing the quantities that would produce the different notes of an octave.[13] Thereby a 'deaf man could put them at any consonance he wished' without hearing anything with regard to the frequency of the strings.[14] For Mersenne, and others in the 17th century, deafmutes raised the question of the mental world of persons deprived of the senses of hearing and speech.[15] Mersenne was also interested in the language of the deaf and dumb.[16] Via a study of the phonetics of speech, and the imitation of human speech by both musical instruments and by animals, Mersenne was led to the whole question of deafmutes and how to communicate with them. His empirical approach rejected the 'widely accepted ancient idea that there was a sympathetic association between the nerves of the ear and the vocal organs, so that the deaf were incurably dumb'.[17] By the 16th century some medical authorities had recognised that the deaf were only dumb because they had never *heard* speech, not because they were incapable of speech itself. Mersenne enthusiastically reported on

the pioneering Spanish work of Pedro Ponce de León in teaching deafmutes to speak.[18]

Communication of and with the deaf

That it was possible to communicate with the congenitally deaf, and even with those deafmute, had already been remarked on in antiquity by Pliny.[19] The possibility of education for and communication with deafmutes is also observed by Augustine, in direct contradiction to his theological views on the position of deafmutes. He mentions the case of a young Milanese man who was deafmute but otherwise fine in body, and well-educated and brought up. Augustine expressly stated that deafness and muteness did not prevent this young man's education, since he spoke with other people by using gestures.[20] Elsewhere Augustine described how the deafmute speak by signs, and not only use signs for visible things, but can also express sounds and tastes through sign language.[21] 'Have you never noticed', he asked, 'how men converse, as it were, with deaf people by gestures and how the deaf in turn use gestures to talk and answer questions, to teach and to make known to each other their wishes ...?'.[22] In the 15th century the humanist Rudolf Agricola mentioned the ability of a deafmute to learn reading and writing as a demonstration of the power of the human spirit: 'I just wish to narrate ... how a person, who was deaf from youth (and consequently also was mute), nevertheless managed to learn to understand everything that someone wrote down'.[23]

The potential of using autochthonous sign language is historically as old as humanity itself, even if structured, regularised and taught sign language is only a phenomenon of the early modern period onward. Evolutionary biology suggests that the development of vocal language was only possible after the human larynx had evolved, some 250,000 years ago, to its present form. Brain development, however, had sped on ahead before the larynx caught up, so that language in the widest sense preceded vocalisation. Sign language then appears to be actually the oldest form of human communication. This theory is backed up by the physiological evidence presented by users of modern sign language, whose hand movements when signing are controlled by the Broca's Region of the brain, normally the language area, and not by the motor control parts of the brain used for other hand movements. It is therefore entirely possible for many different styles and 'grammars' of sign language to have been developed and used by deaf people throughout the ages, in an innate drive for communication. 'Researchers have recently shown us that

---

[10] Sears 1993, 24; Aristotle, *De sensu*, 437a.
[11] Sears 1993, 29: '*Auriculis quasi vestibulo suscepta priore,/ Vox sonat et trahitur interiore domo:/ Sermonis numeros extraque sonancia verba/ Auris, sed ratio significata capit*'; Bernard Silvestris, *Cosmographia*, II. 14. 49-78, ed. P. Dronke, Leiden, 1978, 151-2; also a translation of *Cosmographia* by W. Wetherbee, New York, 1973.
[12] Crombie 1996, 284; Girolamo Cardano, *Opera Omnia*, ii, Lugduni, 1663, 72-3, x, p. 462.
[13] Mersenne 1637
[14] Crombie 1996, 109.
[15] Crombie 1996, 110.
[16] Crombie 1996, 275.
[17] Crombie 1996, 283.

[18] Crombie 1996, 284.
[19] *Historia Naturalis* 35, 21
[20] Werner 1932, 97-8; Augustine, *De quantitate animae, Patrologiae Latinae* (ed. Migne), vol. 32, col. 1052.
[21] Werner 1932, 97-8; Augustine, *De magistro*, cap. 3, *Patrologiae Latinae* (ed. Migne), vol. 32, col. 1197.
[22] Rée 1999, 120; Augustine, *De Magistro*, trans. Robert P. Russell as *The Teacher*, Washington: Catholic University Press of America, 1968, 13.
[23] Werner 1932, 101; Rudolf Agricola, *Inventio dialectica* (my translation from German translation of Latin).

sign language will evolve in deaf children whether or not there is a signing adult teaching them'.[24] With evolutionary and physiological factors indicating the potential of sign language as a feasible communication tool we may assume the existence of such communication methods in past times.

Legal implications of hearing and speech impairments in canon and civil law

Physical impairment under canon law was, of course, an irregularity that prevented the attainment of priesthood - or at least entry into higher orders, the *debilitas corporis* and *defectus scientiae* in the *Decretals* or *'Liber extra'* of Pope Gregory IX.[25] Interestingly, in tests for so-called 'benefit of clergy', where both secular and ecclesiastical courts tried to ascertain if an accused was a clerk and hence subject to the more lenient canon law, the problem of a mute clerk appears. By around 1400 English lawyers tried to find ways, at least hypothetically, to cover all such contingencies, so that the mute clerk was to perform his test in writing, while the blind clerk should speak Latin (but 'from education rather than like an Italian').[26] The issue of how such disabled men could have become clerks in the first place, considering the famous Biblical injunction (Leviticus 21: 17-20) against 'deformed' priests, is quickly clarified: the clerks in question in these legal cases had become disabled *after* their ordination.

Canon law permitted deaf people to marry, by taking their vows through gesturing, as an early form of 'unofficial' sign language - but this applied only to those with acquired deafness and not to the congenitally deaf. Canon law was more concerned about preventing people from marrying who could not fulfill their duty to 'multiply', i.e. those who were frigid, impotent or infertile. For medieval theologians and canonists, such as Gratian's *Decretum*, these were 'disabilities' and impediments to marriage. Opinions were reinforced by the early-13th century *Decretals*, which contained a section 'The Frigid and the Hexed [*Maleficiati*], and Inability to Copulate' (*Decretals*, 4.15). As Noonan says, the 'title dealt with physical disabilities to the contracting of a valid marriage'.[27] Secular law too, for example the 13th-century *Livre de jostice*, from the region of Orléans and influenced by canon law, permitted mute or deaf people to marry, providing they could communicate their intent by signs: 'if they can consent, they can do it; thus if a mute cannot speak, he can just as well make a sign'.[28]

Civil law, which contained elements that had been incorporated from Roman law, also problematised the situation of hearing and speech impaired persons. Here the two main texts of Roman law were the Theodosian[29] and Justinian Codes. In the main, civil law covered the in/ability to give evidence, to make a will or to otherwise participate in legal processes where the ability to communicate meaningfully was paramount.

In the Justinian codes, some distinction was made according to types of hearing and speech impediment. A deaf person could not promise by *stipulatio*, that is an oral contract which only later is written down[30] - although this only applied to those totally deaf and not simply to those who were hard of hearing - but many mute people could conduct all their business affairs as long as they could write.[31] The distinction made between someone congenitally mute and someone with acquired speech impairment in later life meant that those mute from birth were excluded from all personal participation in oral legal transactions, and also excluded from testation. In this sense their legal status was similar to that of children or of mentally impaired persons, who were also deemed incapable (*qui fari non potest*) under the law. Exclusion relates to the restriction imposed on impaired persons to participate fully in public life. The Justinian codes were particularly concerned about impaired people and their ability to make property transactions of various kinds (be it wills, stipulations, promises). According to the *Institutes* (2.10), deaf, mute, or mad persons, as well as women, under-age boys or slaves were all forbidden from appearing as witnesses. Deaf, mute, incurably diseased, insane people and minors had to have curators appointed for them[32] in the same way as children required guardians.[33]

Interestingly, in contrast Jewish Talmudic law expressly forbid the placing of deafmutes with 'idiots' and with those unable to conduct their own affairs, since there was the theoretical possibility of educating the deafmutes and thereby allowing them to acquire reason.[34] But in Roman law, those who became mute in later life, if they could write their own testament, were allowed to make a valid will.[35] Neither mute people nor any others suffering from various impairments could be the legal guardians of minors or of other legally incapable people.[36] But all groups - deaf, mute and blind - could inherit, however. What mattered was not the existence of a certain sensory faculty, nor did a physical or mental impairment automatically exclude a person from legal transactions, but the level of understanding

---

[24] Davis 1995, 18; cf. *New York Times*, 1 Sep 1992, B:6.
[25] Richter and Friedberg 1922 rpt 1955, 1.9.10 and 3.6.1-6.
[26] Swanson 1993, 151; Baker 1997, 330-1. For a selection of law-school texts discussing various scenarios of blind, deaf, or maimed clerks, which more often than not dealt with hypothetical cases for the edification of legal students, cf. J.H. Baker, *The Reports of Sir John Spelman*, Selden Society, vols 93-94, 1976-7, at vol. ii, 328-31.
[27] Noonan, 1965, 289.
[28] Cited by Pfau, *2008*, 118; cf. Louis Nicholas Rapetti (ed.), *Li livres de jostice et de plet, publié pour la première fois d'après le manuscrit unique de la Bibliothèque nationale, Collection de documents inédits sur l'histoire de France, 1. sér. Histoire politique*, Paris, 1850, 183, 23: *'se tés poent consentir, il le poeent; car se li muz ne pot parler, il pot bien*

fere signe'.
[29] Harries and Wood 2010.
[30] O'Neill 1980, 84; cf. Justinian's *Institutes* 3.19.7.
[31] *Institutes* 2.12.3; Werner 1932, 71-3.
[32] *Digest*, III, 3.43; O'Neill 1980, 85.
[33] *Institutes* 1.23.4
[34] Werner 1932, 85 note 2.
[35] *Institutes* II, 12.3, with the fullest text on deafmutes at *Codex Justinianus* 6.22.10; O'Neill 1980, 84.
[36] *Codex Justinianus* 5.68.1 *'qui morbo'*: *'Luminibus captus aut surdus aut mutus aut furiosus aut perpetua valitudine tentus tutelae seu curationis excusationem habent'*.

or 'reason'. This becomes clear in a commentary by the 3rd-century Roman jurist Papinian recorded in Justinian's *Digest* (37.3), where the deaf, mute or blind were able to make inheritance claims if they understood the legality of the transaction[37] - therefore comprehension was the defining criterion, not the ability to speak, hear or see.

The so-called barbarian laws, with some influence of the Theodosian code, primarily mention deafness or speech impairment in the context of compensation schemes for different injuries. The Frisian laws, compiled between 785 and 803, appear to be the only ones that include a tariff specifically for muteness, fining the culprit 18 *solidi* (i.e. 18% of the wergild commonly set at 100 *solidi*) for striking a blow that renders the victim dumb.[38] The tariff scheme in the *Lex Saxonum* of c. 802 combined a carefully thought-out hierarchy of what the injury or loss of a specific body part meant, in terms of its impact on the overall physiological functioning of a person. For example, losing the thumb impairs ability to grip and is therefore rated higher than loss of a finger. Such schemes provide us with some interesting examples of the culturally-specific perception of physical impairment. Sensory impairment, here in the case of blindness and deafness, is rated as severely as the killing of a noble woman - perhaps connected with the notion of the severely impaired person as occupying a liminal territory, existing between health and illness, life and death.[39] In the *Leges Henrici Primi* (c.93,37) this concept is also encountered, where the relatively high compensation of 100 shillings is to be paid in cases of neck injury severe enough so that the person affected 'yet remains alive though thus incapacitated'.

With Anglo-Saxon England, in the 9th-century law code of King Alfred, we are closer to the old Roman laws than to tariff schemes with regard to hearing and speech impairments. 'If anyone is born dumb or deaf, so that he cannot deny or confess his sins, his father shall pay compensation for his misdeeds'.[40] Here the congenitally deaf-mute are exempt from punishment, yet the otherwise adult but impaired man is treated as a child under the law. The concept of *unmagum*, that is of not being capable, not being able to do something, is repeated in Alfred 17 with regard to dependent persons. Frederick Attenborough had translated this passage to infer children (or other) helpless persons,[41] but in the light of the use of similar wording (*unmagum*) here as only a few articles earlier (in Alfred 14: *ne maege*) it is more likely that, as Sally Crawford has suggested,[42] the notion of *unmagum/ne maege* implies a

more general state of not being capable, hence coming close to the modern concept of 'disability'. Nordic cultural mentalities found their way into the laws of Canute promulgated in England: here people were excluded from burial in consecrated ground if they had not been able to recite the Creed and the Paternoster, something it is likely will have affected those who were congenitally deaf or speech impaired.

Bracton

Infantilisation and abrogation of the legal rights normally accorded to non-impaired adults begin to emerge as the main themes of legal notions. They come to be fully, even verbosely expressed by the English jurist Bracton. Jumping ahead to the 13th century, we find here a more or less complete reception of the legal restrictions placed on deaf and mute people that the Justinian code had contained:

> There is also an exception arising from the person of the demandant if he is naturally deaf and dumb.

Being born deaf and dumb is a natural defect 'as where one is born deaf and dumb, so that he cannot speak or hear at all'.[43] As in the Justinian code this is regarded as something separate from just hard of hearing or having a minor speech impediment:

> One naturally deaf and dumb cannot acquire because he cannot consent, because he is completely unable to hear the words of the stipulator, and since he cannot hear or speak at all, he cannot express his will and consent either by words or signs. 'Naturally', I say, that is, from birth, as one speaks of a blind man who was blind from birth, for if this comes about accidentally, there must be an enquiry as to what he was like before the accident, because if at first he could speak and hear and consent [and] acquires, by himself or by a procurator, he retains what he had acquired, though he does not easily transfer it to another.[44]

So if sensory disability is not congenital but acquired (accidentally), then the law needs to find out what communication abilities and what level of rationality a person had before becoming disabled. In terms of ownership, the congenitally deaf and dumb are treated like minors. Bracton had addressed the issue in another passage:

> To whom the right may descend.

> And so of one naturally deaf and dumb, if he cannot hear or speak at all, but if he can, though only with difficulty, the same may be said, that he may acquire

[37] Mommsen and Krueger (eds), 1985 at vol. 3, 277-8.
[38] Oliver 2001, 96 and 257.
[39] Cf Metzler 2006, 31-2 for an exploration of the theme of the impaired person being in limbo.
[40] Alfred 14, in Attenborough 1922 rpt 2000, 71.
[41] Attenborough 1922 rpt 2000, 73.
[42] Sally Crawford 2010. An alternative lexeme in old English inferring 'disability' in the widest sense is *unhal* (that which is un-whole), found in the Laws of Cnud and Ethelred, also in a prayer to St Margaret, which asks to prevent the birth of a disabled child (i.e. a child that is not crippled, deaf, blind, dumb or mentally impaired). However it is notable that *unhal* is not used in Old English to describe the wounds, infirmities or torture marks of the martyrs and saints - the linguistic

differentiation delineating a difference in causal 'types' of disability? See Metzler (forthcoming 2013), 'Indiscriminate healing miracles in decline: how social realities affect religious perception', in M. Mesley and L.E. Wilson (eds) *Contextualizing Medieval Miracles*, for the theory that saintly bodies come to stand in juxtaposition to the disabilities of 'ordinary' people.
[43] Woodbine and Thorne 1977, vol. 4, 309.
[44] Woodbine and Thorne 1977, vol. 4, p. 309.

and retain and transfer to others, because such persons may consent, at least by signs and a nod.[45]

Therefore someone only partially deaf or mildly speech-impaired can enter legal transactions by using (unofficial and unspecified) sign language, although Bracton repeated the problems of a dumb person not saying the required words[46] and of deaf mutes not hearing them, making the provision to use 'tutors or curators' as is done for minors.

If a parcener is deaf or dumb.

In the case of congenital deafness a parcener (that is a partner or person having a share in land or property with another) is treated like a minor, 'but if the deafness arises from an accident or if he is dumb and deafness does not ensue, a period of time must be awaited if there is hope of recovery'.[47]

What kind of seisin bars the assise.

In connection with the ability to partake in an assise, being deaf and mute is termed a 'defect of nature or sense'. Apart from that Bracton repeats yet again the distinction between congenital deafness and muteness, and those simply hard of hearing or with a speech impediment. 'But if the deafness is accidental, the assise does not fall but must be postponed until the tenant's condition is improved'.[48] And once more the deaf and dumb are compared to the insane.

Who cannot stipulate.

This passage is again an amalgamation and reworking of several passages from the Justinian code. A speech impaired person cannot utter the necessary words, nor can a deafmute, unless both parties agree on using 'a nod or a writing'.[49] The by now familiar distinction between the hard of hearing and the 'stone-deaf' is made yet again. Interestingly, the reasons why lunatics and children cannot stipulate are separated out from those why the deafmute cannot do so - for once there is a clear separation between deaf/mutes on the one hand and lunatics/infants on the other.

Excuses for not putting in a claim.

However, like in many medieval texts, things are not as straightforward or neatly consistent as they seem. In this passage concerning excuses for not putting in a claim,

Bracton does lump 'idiots and those born deaf and dumb and the like' into the same bracket, since those persons 'lack reason',[50] while allowing for this condition to change only for the madmen and children, but not for the congenitally deafmute. If we take this particular passage in isolation the impression emerges that, according to Bracton, the mental abilities of deafmutes are permanently fixed below the required level of rationality.

Other jurists

In France, Bracton's contemporary Philippe de Beaumanoir, whose *Coutumes de Beauvaisis* were composed around 1283, made similar distinctions between the totally deaf and the hard of hearing with regard to the validity of legal agreements:

> because a mute person cannot make an agreement since he cannot speak, and an agreement cannot be made without words; nor can a deaf person, since he cannot hear the agreement, but here we understand deaf people who never hear anything, because a person who hears when you shout can make an agreement
>
> (*car li mus ne puet fere convenance pour ce qu'il ne puet parler, car convenance ne se puet fere sans parole; ne li sours pour ce qu'il ne puet oïr la convenance, mes ce entendons nous des sours qui n'oient nule goute, car ci qui oit par haut parler puet bien fere convenance.*)[51]

Thus yet again the overarching importance of spoken language, the relic of the primal heard word, is brought to the fore when it came to the treatment of deaf and mute persons under the law.

Another form of excluding the mentally and physically impaired may be found in English law of the 13th century (Whittaker's *The Mirror of Justices*) where the following kinds of people are forbidden from becoming judges: 'women ... serfs, and those under the age of twenty-one, open lepers, idiots, attorneys, lunatics, deaf mutes, those excommunicated by a bishop, criminal persons'.[52] And in Germany too, the *Burggrafenrecht* of Cologne excluded deaf and speech impaired persons from holding any judicial office,[53] while in southern Germany the *Brünner Schöffenbuch* stated that a judge was not allowed to be lame in hands or feet, nor blind, nor mute.[54] Such notions were carried forward into the Golden Bull of emperor Charles IV of 1356/7, where chapter 25 deals with the exclusion of the son of an elector from primogeniture if he is mentally afflicted, dumb or otherwise visibly impaired.[55]

---

[45] Woodbine and Thorne 1977, vol. 4, p. 178.
[46] The importance of 'getting it right' in spoken language is of course vital within a culture that to a great extent uses oral legal representation: the accuser had to make their claim audibly and correctly, using the right words. In the *Sachsenspiegel* one finds similar caution concerning correct wordage, so that a man who stammers and 'mis-says' his claim has to have a chance to have it said correctly: '*Der stamerende man, ab her misspricht, muz sich wol erholen. Versumet her ouch ienen man, des vorspreche her iz, der muz sich wol erholen mit eime anderen vorsprechen*' (*Sachsenspiegel* Landrecht 1.LXI.3, Ebel, 1999, 64).
[47] Woodbine and Thorne 1977, vol. 4, p. 339.
[48] Woodbine and Thorne 1977, vol. 3, 300.
[49] Woodbine and Thorne 1977, vol. 2, 286.

[50] Woodbine and Thorne 1977, vol. 4, 356.
[51] English translation by Pfau 2008, 119; cf. Salmon 1970-74, vol. 2, chp. 34, § 1061.
[52] Rushton 1996, 47.
[53] Drüppel 1981, 86.
[54] Drüppel 1981, 87.
[55] Hergemöller 1994, 5.

In the *Sachsenspiegel* there has been a shift in focus, and here it is not the deafmutes of Roman law who are excluded, but 'dwarfs' and 'cripples', presumably since by the early 13th century property and tenancy were linked, at least theoretically, with knights' fees and military duties so that the more obvious physical impairments that could prevent a person from performing feudal dues may have been significant. This begs the question why other forms of physical impairment, such as the sensory impairments of deaf, mute and blind, so often encountered in the Roman texts, were not regarded as inhibiting someone's capability of performing military or knightly duties. Interestingly, at least one ruler of a medieval kingdom, John the Blind (1296-1346), duke of Luxembourg and king of Bohemia, did not let his 'disability' (he was blind from 1340) get in the way of military campaigning - he died, famously, leading his troops in the charge at the battle of Crécy.[56]

The connection with feudal dues only becomes apparent in Book I.4 of the *Sachsenspiegel*:

> A child born dumb, blind, or lacking hand or foot is a legitimate heir according to the territorial law but not according to feudal law. If he has been granted a fief before this [disability] occurred, then he forfeits nothing. A leper cannot succeed to feudal tenancy or hereditary property, but if he was invested before the illness and becomes ill afterwards, then he does not forfeit it.
>
> (*Wirt ouch ein kint stum geboren adir handelos, vuzeloz adir blint, daz ist wol erbe zu lantrechte unde en iz nicht lenerbe. Hat ez abir len entphangen, er ez wurde alsus, daz en verluset ez damete nicht. Der maselsuchtige man entphet weder len noch erbe. Hat er ez abir entphangen er der suche, her behelt ez unde erbit ez alse ein ander man.*)[57]

We can compare this distinction between two types of landholding in the *Sachsenspiegel* to the distinction given by Bracton of legal ownership - *proprietas* and possession. The right to property is available to all, 'whether he is a minor or of full age, a male or a female, a madman or a fool, as an idiot, one who is deaf and dumb',[58] but possession does not automatically follow.

Finally with regard to the legal 'problem' of deaf and mute persons, one must consider how medieval jurisprudence dealt with the theoretical inculpability of these people whilst confronted with the factual criminal deeds, including homicide, of such sensory disabled people. According to modern notions of legal culpability deaf and mute persons, unlike the insane, might be deemed fully responsible for their criminal actions, but in the Middle Ages 'the absence of methods for teaching them [meant] they must often have

had little understanding of law and morality'.[59] Looking at cases from English 13th-century documents regarding homicides it appears that since the speech-impaired were unable to plead mercy or pardon 'they were treated as being incapable of defending themselves and so of being judged'.[60] There is a case in the Close Rolls for 1231-34 of one mute man, who knew about taking church sanctuary after he had killed another man. He remained in church for eight and a half years, when Henry III allowed the abbot of Shireburn to take this man to his abbey and keep him there 'provided he never went beyond its walls'.[61] There is a hint here concerning the ambiguity of that man's culpability. In a late-13th century case of homicide from the Calendar of Patent Rolls, 1292-1301 (no. 250), the king's pardon might be obtained for a deaf-mute culprit.[62] Because being deaf and mute is so easy to fake by pretenders, people start treating the notion of inculpability with suspicion. There is anecdotal evidence that by the 17th century purportedly mute people were put to torture to get them to cry out in pain, so as to prove they were not really speechless.[63]

Philosophical and theological approaches

Laws then are part of the cultural assumptions about the difference and inferiority of a person's disability that may lead to exclusion in daily life. But legal concepts are only part of wider normative forces. As an example, the notion of the innocence, therefore of the inability to be sinful, and in legal parlance the criminal inculpability of the deaf, the mute - and the mentally disabled - can be taken further into the realm of philosophy and theology.

This was succinctly expressed in the *Ethics* of Peter Abelard. Writing before 1140 he stated: 'Of [sin] small children and of course insane people are untouched; because they, who also lack reason, have no merits and therefore nothing is counted as sin for them'.[64] We have seen that legally the congenitally deaf were sometimes categorised with children and the insane.[65] These cannot sin, they are innocent, but that is precisely because they lack reason, which in other respects is one of the defining characteristics of a human being - one need only think of the Aristotelian 'rational animal' that is the definition of the human. In the 13th century Thomas Aquinas, that great synthesiser of Aristotelian philosophy and Catholic theology, had responded to the argument that the mentally impaired were like beasts by pointing out:

> Madmen and imbeciles lack the use of reason accidentally, i.e. through some impediment in a bodily organ; but not like irrational animals through want of a rational soul.

---

[56] Discussing the (in)significance of John the Blind: Singer 2011, 101-3; Wheatley 2010, 194-204.
[57] *The Saxon Mirror*, Book I.4, Debozy, 199, 69-70 and *Sachsenspiegel* Landrecht 1.IV, Ebel, 1999, 32.
[58] Woodbine and Thorne 1977, vol. 2, 24.

[59] Hurnard 1996, 169.
[60] *Ibid.*
[61] *Ibid.*
[62] *Ibid.*
[63] McKenzie 2005.
[64] Luscombe 1971, 56; cf. Porter 2000.
[65] On this subject see also Metzler 2010, 197-217.

(furiosi vel amentes carent usu rationis per accidens, scilicet propter aliquod impedimentum organi corporalis: non autem propter defectum animae rationalis, sicut bruta animalia.)[66]

The irrationality of the insane, and by implication of the deaf, was therefore due to physical causes, not spiritual, and hence the insane and the deaf could be saved. Aquinas further elaborated on the topic, by distinguishing between four types of mental incapacity: those who were congenitally insane and never had any 'lucid moments', those who had fallen from sanity into insanity, those who were congenitally insane yet could have lucid moments, and finally those 'others who, although not altogether sane, yet can use their reason so far as to think about their salvation, and understand the power of the sacrament'.[67] By the later Middle Ages such philosophical concepts could be expanded into religious thought (and perhaps practice). Regarding the ceremony of the Eucharist, a late medieval notion held that animals, infidels and the irrational or unthinking cannot experience the Eucharist properly.[68] Thomas Aquinas had held that those who were in his first category of irrationality, the congenitally afflicted without lucid moments, should not receive the Eucharist, although if a person had at any time in their life been capable of rationality, then they could receive (and continue to receive) the Eucharist.[69] Based on the medieval normative texts I have discussed, by the 'irrational and unthinking' one must also understand the congenitally deaf/mute. According to this view, such people cannot benefit from the religious experience offered, which leads one to ponder the question as to whether in actuality they may even have been excluded from participation in the Eucharist. And lest we forget the importance of hearing, let us remind ourselves that in religious practice confession was to be heard, with one participant speaking, the other hearing - never at any stage was confession something you could 'do in writing', let alone remotely, but always something to be performed, if not face to face then mouth to ear (this is evident in the title alone of H. C. Lea's 1896 book, *A History of Auricular Confession*).[70] The primacy of hearing is expressed in a sermon for Easter Sunday by John Felton, parish priest of St Mary Magdalene, Oxford from 1397 to 1434, and famous as a preacher. The author states 'we should know how all man's senses are mistaken about the sacrament, all except hearing'.[71] In an allegory, the sermon writer explains that the five senses are like the messengers of the soul, but sight, smell, taste and touch are only capable of sensing the material aspects, while hearing alone recognises the divine within the ordinary 'bread' of the sacrament, based on the infamous passage in Romans 10:17 on faith coming through hearing.

The contradiction between medieval notions of the deaf as innocent and free of sin on the one hand, while on the other hand their inability to hear the word of God rendered them incapable of becoming true Christians, raises some interesting questions. Simply put, like most societies, medieval society was also not free from inherent contradictions. Some elements of society (theologians and their theory) could describe the inability to gain the faith by the deaf, while other elements (civil lawyers, based partly on the earlier 'barbarian' laws as well as Roman legal traditions) could emphasize the lack of culpability. And sometimes these contradictions may be encountered in the writings of one single individual, for instance none other than Augustine in two of his texts, both cited above, expounds these two different viewpoints: while in one text he stated that congenitally deafmute or blind children suffered even more than their parents due to their inability to acquire the faith, in other texts he asserted that education of, and communication with, deafmutes was a distinct possibility by employing sign language.[72] However, one may argue that overall, late antique and medieval philosophical and religious notions underpinned the primacy of language and ensured the relegation of the deaf and mute to a dubious status, ambiguously sharing qualities of both rational man and the dumb beasts.

Linguistic deafness

The primacy of spoken/heard language is also reflected in language itself. *Daffe/daft* for 'deaf' in Middle English becomes *daft* for 'stupid' in modern English. Modern English 'deaf' starts off as Old English *déaf*. Modern German *taub* has the same root as *toben* (raging, raving madness) and *dumm* (stupid) via *toub/toup* in Middle High German, which has meanings of deaf, not hearing, not feeling/sensing, foolish. Modern German makes a connection between *taub* as deaf and *betäuben* 'to stun', so both *taub* and *betäuben* relate to desensitising, *stumpfsinnig machen*. The deaf person is therefore linguistically not far removed from the senseless person. Words for deafness are linguistically related to insanity, imbecility and irrationality - the very lexemes themselves can express the primacy of spoken language.

However, linguistic deafness can occasionally function as disobedience. In the German language there are some further interesting meanings and associations of the expression *hören*. A serf or dependent peasant was referred to as *hörig*, somebody who has to hear (and listen and obey) the words of his lord and master. The word for belonging,

---

[66] English: Thomas Aquinas, *Summa theologica*, trans. Fathers of the English Dominican Province, Westminster: Christian Classics, 1981, 5 vols, at vol. 4, 2402; Latin: Thomas Aquinas, *Summa Theologiae*, ed. James J. Cunningham, London: Blackfriars, 1964, 60 vols, at vol. 57, 120, q 68, 12.

[67] English: Thomas Aquinas, *Summa theologica*, trans. Fathers of the English Dominican Province, Westminster: Christian Classics, 1981, 5 vols, at vol. 4, 2402; Latin: '*nulla habentes lucida intervalla. ... Quidam vero sunt qui, etsi non omnino sanae mentis existent, in tantum tamen ratione utuntur quod possunt de sua salute cogitare, et intelligere sacramenti virtutem*', Thomas Aquinas, *Summa Theologiae*, ed. James J. Cunningham, London: Blackfriars, 1964, 60 vols, at vol. 57, 118-20, q 68, 12.

[68] Rubin 1991, 67.

[69] Pfau 2008, 82-3.

[70] Lea 1896.

[71] Wenzel 2008, 139; translated from Oxford, Bodleian Library, MS Bodley 187, fols 47ra-49ra.

[72] For negative view: Werner 1932, 74; cf. Augustine, *Contra Julian. Pelagian.*, III, cap. 4, *Patrologiae Latinae* (ed. Migne), vol. 44, col. 707. For positive view: Werner 1932, 97-8; Augustine, *De quantitate animae*, *Patrologiae Latinae* (ed. Migne), vol. 32, col. 1052; and Augustine, *De magistro*, cap. 3, *Patrologiae Latinae* (ed. Migne), vol. 32, col. 1197.

as in being a possession, is *gehören*, ge+hören, so he who has to listen is simultaneously he who belongs. Obedience (*gehorchen*) is linguistically linked to hearing (*Gehör geben, zuhören*). The *Hörige* serf literally belongs (*gehört*) to his lord, whose commands he hears and has to act upon. In that sense the deaf person is the legally disobedient person - think of modern people pretending to be deaf so as to avoid something. Deliberate deafness circumvents the niceties of polite behaviour, allows one to blatantly ignore unwelcome social demands. One cannot emphasise enough how hearing and listening have historically been associated with obedience and possession. But with greater literacy and greater use of texts for administration, the formerly close link between hearing (*hören*) and being owned (*gehören*) remains solely as a linguistic fossil.

This essay started with the description of an image *of* a hearing-impaired person, but I wish to conclude with some tentative thoughts on the seeing - and understanding - of images *by* hearing-impaired persons. The point can be made that although the deaf may not have been able to hear, especially not to hear the word of God, they were nevertheless perfectly capable of seeing images or reading. However these capacities only apply to such people who became deaf later in life, to persons with acquired deafness rather than to the congenitally deaf who have been the main subject of this essay. The congenitally deaf would not have been able to gain the 'cultural baggage' necessary to interpret images in the first place, never mind learning

to read, for without such cultural conditioning how do you approach images? Any modern reader who has ever tried 'reading' imagery in a medieval church will recognise this problem. Ask someone unfamiliar with the oral story associated with a visual image, such as a small child, and, for example, scenes of Noah building the Ark might be described simply as 'man with axe in front of shed', but only prior knowledge of the story of Noah allows the viewer to recognise the 'type' as Noah's Ark scenes and interpret them accordingly. In fact, this very point is made in a 13th-century source from the miracles of St Louis, where a deafmute man is described as 'participating' in church ritual only because of social habit, copying what other people do, or from an innate notion of what is 'right' and 'proper', but without truly 'understanding':

> he did not know or understand anything about God and his saints. However, when he was with [his adoptive family] ... he had often seen them go to church and pray there and have devotion, and kneel and raise their eyes with their hands joined together and raised to the sky. For that reason he now went to the church [of Saint Denis], but not because he knew what a church was or what devotion was ... And thus it happened that when the blessed king was entombed, because he saw the other men kneeling and praying at the tomb, he too knelt and joined his hands without knowing what he was doing.[73]

---

[73] Farmer 2009, 204.

67

Bibliography

Attenborough, F.L. (ed. and trans.) 1922 rpt 2000. *The Laws of the Earliest English Kings*, Cambridge: rpt Felinfach.

Baker, J.H. 1977. *The Reports of Sir John Spelman*, Selden Society, vol. 94.

Crawford, S. 2010. 'Differentiation in the later Anglo-Saxon burial ritual on the basis of mental or physical impairment: a documentary perspective', in A. Cherryson and J. Buckberry, *Burial in Later Anglo-Saxon England, c. AD 650-1100*, 93-102. Oxford: Oxbow Books.

Crombie, A.C. 1996. *Science, Art and Nature in Medieval and Modern Thought*, London & Rio Grande: Hambledon press

Davis, L.J. 1995. *Enforcing Normalcy: Disability, Deafness, and the Body*, London and New York: Verso Books.

Debozy, M. (trans.) 1999. *The Saxon Mirror*, Philadelphia: University of Pennsylvania Press.

Drüppel, H. 1981. *Judex civitatis: zur Stellung des Richters in der hoch- und spätmittelalterlichen Stadt*, Cologne: Forschungen zur deutschen Rechtsgeschichte 12.

Ebel, F. (ed.) 1999. *Sachsenspiegel. Landrecht und Lehnrecht*, Stuttgart: Reclam Philipp Jun.

Farmer, S. 2009. 'A deaf-mute's story', in M. Rubin (ed.), *Medieval Christianity in Practice*, 203-208. Princeton, NJ: Princeton University Press.

Fischer, B., Gribomont, I., Sparks, H.F.D. and Thiele W., (eds) 1994. *Biblia Sacra iuxta Vulgatem Versionem*, 4th ed. Stuttgart: Hendrickson Publishers Inc.

Harries, J. and Wood, I. (eds) 2010. *The Theodosian Code: Studies in the Imperial Law of Late Antiquity*, 2nd ed. London: Cornell University Press.

Hergemöller, B.-U. (ed.) 1994. *Randgruppen der spätmittelalterlichen Gesellschaft*, 2nd ed. Warendorf: Fahlbusch.

Hurnard, N.D. 1996. *The King's Pardon for Homicide before A.D. 1307*, Oxford: Clarendon Press.

Luscombe, D.E. (ed.) 1971. *Peter Abelard's Ethics*, Oxford: Clarendon Press.

Lea, H.C. 1896. *A History of Auricular Confession and Indulgences in the Latin church*, 2 vols. Philadelphia: Lea Brothers and Co.

McKenzie, A. 2005. '"This Death Some Strong and Stout Hearted Man Doth Choose": the practice of *peine forte et dure* in seventeenth- and eighteenth-century England', *Law and History Review*, **23 (2)**, 279-313.

Mersenne, M. 1637. *Harmonie Universelle*, Paris: Pierre Ballard.

Metzler, I. 2006. *Disability in Medieval Europe: Thinking about Physical Impairment during the High Middle Ages, c.1100-1400*, Routledge Studies in Medieval Religion and Culture 5. London and New York: Routledge.

Metzler, I. 2010. 'Afterword', in W.J. Turner (ed), *Madness in Medieval Law and Custom*, 197-218. Later Medieval Europe 6, Leiden: Brill.

Mommsen, T. and Krueger, P. (eds) 1985. *The Digest of Justinian*, 4 vols. Philadelphia, PA: University of Philadelphia Press.

Noonan, J.T. 1965. *Contraception: a History of its Treatment by the Catholic Theologians and Canonists*, Cambridge, MA: Belknap Press of Harvard University Press.

Oliver, L. 2001. *The Body Legal in Barbarian Law*, Toronto, Buffalo and London: University of Toronto Press.

O'Neill, Y.V. 1980. *Speech and Speech Disorders in Western Thought before 1600* (Contributions in Medical History, Number 3), Westport, CT and London: Greenwood Press.

Pfau, A.N. 2008. *Madness in the Realm: Narratives of Mental Illness in Late Medieval France*, PhD diss., University of Michigan.

Porter, J. 2000. 'Responsibility, passion, and sin: a reassessment of Abelard's ethics', *The Journal of Religious Ethics*, **28(3)**, 367-394.

Rée, J. 1999. *I See a Voice: a Philosophical History of Language, Deafness and the Senses*, London: Flamingo.

Richter, E.L. and Friedberg, E. (eds) 1881. *Corpus Iuris Canonici II*, Leipzig: Bernhard Tauchnitz, rpt 1955 Graz: Akademische Druck-U. Verlagsanstalt.

Rubin, M. 1991. *Corpus Christi: the Eucharist in Late Medieval culture*, Cambridge: Cambridge University Press.

Rushton, P. 1996. 'Idiocy, the family and the community in early modern north-east England', in D. Wright and A. Digby (eds), *From Idiocy to Mental Deficiency: Historical Perspectives on People with Learning Disabilities*, 44-64. London and New York: Routledge.

Salmon, A. (ed). 1970-74. *Phillipe de Beaumanoir: Coutumes de Beauvaisis*, Paris: A. Picard et Fils.

Sears, E. 1993. 'Sensory perception and its metaphors in the time of Richard of Fournival', in W.F. Bynum and R. Porter (eds), *Medicine and the Five Senses*, 17-39. Cambridge: Cambridge University Press.

Seidenspinner-Núñez, D. (trans.) 1998. *The writings of Teresa de Cartagena*, Cambridge: D.S. Brewer.

Singer, J. 2011. *Blindness and Therapy in Late Medieval French and Italian Poetry*, Gallica 20. Cambridge: D.S. Brewer.

Swanson, R.N. 1993. *Church and Society in Late Medieval England*, Oxford: Oxford University Press.

Wenzel, S. (trans) 2008. *Preaching in the Age of Chaucer: Selected Sermons in Translation*, Washingon DC: The Catholic University of America Press.

Werner, H. 1932. *Geschichte des Taubstummenproblems bis ins 17. Jahrhundert*, Jena: G. Fisher.

Wheatley, E. 2010. *Stumbling Blocks before the Blind: Medieval Constructions of a Disability*, Ann Arbor: the University of Michigan Press.

Woodbine, G.E (ed.) and Thorne S.E. (trans.) 1977. *Bracton on the Laws and Customs of England*, 4 vols. Cambridge, MA: Belknap Press of Harvard University Press.

Woolgar, C.M. 2006. *The Senses in Late Medieval England*, New Haven and London: Yale University Press.

Chapter 8
Leprosy, Lepers and Leper-houses: between Human Law and God's Law (6th-15th centuries)[1]

Damien Jeanne

To Julia Milched

Introduction

In the very first pages of his famous opus *The Waning of the Middle Ages* (1919), Johan Huizinga (1872-1945) emphasized the paradoxical situation of those who are weak and harshly treated, but are at the same time protected:

> The contrast of cruelty and of pity recurs at every turn in the manners and customs of the Middle Ages. On the one hand, the sick, the poor, the insane, are objects of that deeply moved pity, born of a feeling of fraternity akin to that which is so strikingly expressed in modern Russian literature; on the other hand, they are treated with incredible hardness or cruelly mocked.[2]

In a more recent book, Robert Ian Moore also insisted on that ambiguous perception of lepers, 'objects of admiration and even envy, as well as terror'. He also underlined the fact that lepers 'constituted a quasi-religious order':

> For Christians the living death of leprosy was an object of admiration and even envy, as well as terror. The leper had been granted the special grace of entering upon payment for his sins in this life, and could therefore look forward to earlier redemption in the next. (…) Like hermits and monks lepers were often called *pauperes Christi*, and the strict rules governing the conduct of leper houses were in part a reflection of the idea that lepers constituted a quasi-religious order.[3]

As for David Nirenberg, his view of the leper is far too one-sided: 'The leper was a heretic or an unrepentant sinner and should be separated from communion with society'.[4] On the other hand, one might try to improve the meaning of 'the ritual of physical isolation of lepers from society'.[5] Leprosy was the sinner's retribution and at the same time a divine election predestining the religious condition.[6]

There was no cure for leprosy in the Middle Ages. In some cases the disease induces severe disability. It disfigures and conveys a number of stereotypes, leading to a loss of identity, of reputation.[7] We should identify two views of leprosy: a disease oscillating on the one hand between a curse (a distinctive sign of sin, leading to a loss of one's reputation) and on the other hand, a blessing - a sign of divine election - a gain in reputation. Squeezed between being condemned by a disease contracted as punishment for their sins and being redeemed by their sufferings, medieval lepers were humiliated yet glorious.

Either way, individuals lost their identity to become mere patients: as a result, lepers were separated, sacred beings, some of whom lived together in well-regulated brotherhoods. The definition of the sacred, borrowed from the works of René Girard, starts with the assumption that sacredness and violence are to be united, within a *Societas christiana* regarded at the time as a society of sacrifice.[8] Michel Foucault had indeed perceived it as such with 'the shepherd's paradox: sacrifice of one individual for the whole, sacrifice of the whole to save the individual, a paradox definitely at the heart of the Christian perspective of priesthood'.[9]

François-Olivier Touati and Marcia Kupfer mention the ambiguous nature of lepers in medieval society, an ambiguity which placed them between sin and redemption. The diseased person embodied at one and the same time the sign of divine mercy and the brand of the offence leading on to conversion.[10] It seems to me that this ambivalence corresponds to the *token of sacredness* as defined by William Robertson Smith (1894), Émile Durkheim (1912),[11] and René Girard (1972):

1. The pure and the impure make up the obverse and reverse sides of a same coin, of sacredness.[12]

2. Sacredness and violence are inseparable.[13] Leprosy is deadly. The individual stricken by that disease is dramatically affected in his mobility and consequently in his ability to provide for himself. Should he survive for a while, he is likely to become a burden, for leprosy does not kill in one blow. Lesions over-infected by environmental bacteria suppurate and become gangrenous, septicemia leading to death.[14] Death is undoubtedly the worst form of violence perpetrated against Man, not counting the stages of physical degradation lepers go through. Death

[1] Translation Geneviève Cornevin-Ferrari.
[2] Huizinga 1924, 26.
[3] Moore 2007, 57; Moore 2012, 6, 64, 108-09, 218, 279.
[4] Nirenberg 1996, 57.
[5] Nirenberg 1996, 57.
[6] Legrand 1901, XXVII; Touati 1998, 244, 237, 401, 404-06; Kupfer 2003, 137; Rawcliffe 2006, 57, 128-33.

[7] Gauvard 2010, 733-34.
[8] Girard 2006, 34.
[9] Foucault 2004,132-34; Foucault 2012, 251, 254; Dalarun 2012, 289.
[10] Touati 2000, 188-90; Kupfer 2003, 137.
[11] Robertson Smith 1889, 152; Durkheim 1912, 65.
[12] Durkheim 1912, 588.
[13] Girard 2006, 34, 52-3.
[14] Pattyn *et al* 1981, 49.

was regarded as a stain. By creating a separate category, churchmen drove away the impurity of leprosy.

These two proposals may provide an explanatory framework coherent with the oscillating, dual behaviours, and the other 'contradictory overlapping' mentioned by François-Olivier Touati.[15] Isolation was the sign of sacredness becoming effective through such rites as the ceremony marking the admittance to the leper-house or the medical examination undergone from the 1260s onward.[16] Since the origins of Christianity, lepers have offered a permanently ambivalent figure[17] going hand in hand with the image of the Christian body.[18]

12th century doctors were well aware of the pathology inherent in leprosy and could not fail to make the right diagnosis, as is shown in the palaeopathologies studied in European archaeological research work.[19] Leprosy is infectious, but it is not that contagious, even if there is a genetic hereditary disposition.[20]

How can we explain the recourse to isolation, albeit relative, when Christianity established, as early as the 3rd century AD, a form of priestly government based on individual salvation and collective charity?

The isolation of lepers: laws against vagrancy?

Protecting the most vulnerable, lepers in particular, became the rule with the spread of Christianity in Gaul. The canon laws passed by the Councils of Orléans (549) and Tours (567) recommended that bishops, priests and parishioners fed lepers and the poor to prevent begging.[21] Begging meant getting exposed to possible acts of violence from the population. To that end, Henry II Plantagenet ordered his officers, in a diploma dated c.1161, to compensate for the harm done to the lepers of Dieppe[22] and to their servants. In order to maintain the peace, the king's provisions for lepers had to be sufficient to prevent disorder-inducing begging.[23] In his *Chronique*, Gilbert Chandelier, a monk

of Saint-Pierre de Préaux in the 12th century, justified the existence of a group of lepers of St Giles in Pont-Audemer by a triple exigency: caring, a monastic way of life, and protecting lepers from beggary.[24] According to the chronicle of the Île-Dieu, Gautier Maloiseau gathered all the lepers of Bolbec,[25] endowing them with enough to prevent them from leaving the place and setting them a rule of life containing four degrees of perfection.[26]

Avoiding contact with the crowd in order to beg seemed to be a legislative invariant.[27] From the 6th to the 15th century, a constant can be seen: lepers' vagrancy was improper.[28] Their uncontrolled vagrancy was *de facto* condemned.[29]

The only solution to vagrancy seemed be to deal food out to the lepers. At the Salle-aux-Puelles, the 1249 book of regulations maintained the previous habits. The archbishop of Rouen, Eudes Rigaud († 1276), emphasized communal life, daily bread, and wine in sufficient quantity.[30] The power of pastoral care was in the flock's salvation which was obtained first of all through subsistence allowances. The shepherd, in this case the bishop or the priest, fed the leper himself, as Jesus fed men.[31] Michel Foucault defines pastoral power as a power of care.[32] The aim of leper-houses fitted this purpose: to care for body and soul within a regular institution. If they were not inside, the leper received neither attention, nor salvation.

[15] Touati 1998, 190, 703, 714, 729.
[16] Durkheim 1912, 428; Touati 1998, 733.
[17] Le Blévec 2000, 835.
[18] Sot 1985, 12-4.
[19] Touati, 1998, 128-38; Ortner 2002, 73-7.
[20] Touati 1998, 52, 139-51; Touati 2000, 179-201; Demaitre 2007, 131, 155-59; Mira *et al* 2003, 412-15; Ranque 2008, 491-97.
[21] '21. *Et licet propitio Deo omnium Domini sacerdotum vel quorumcumque haec cura possit esse fidelium, ut egentibus necessaria debeant ministrare, specialiter tamen de leprosis id pietatis causa convenit, ut unusquisque episcoporum, quos incolas hanc infirmitatem incurrisse tam territorii sui quam civitatis agnoverit, de domo ecclesiae juxta possibilitatem victui et vestitui necessaria subministret, ut non his desit misericordia cura, quos per duram infirmitatem intolerabilis constringit inopia*' (Gaudemet and Basdevant 1989, 316-17): '5. *Ut unaquaeque civitas pauperes et egenos incolas alimentis congruentibus pascat secundum vires; ut tam vicani prebyteri quam cives omnes suum pauperem pascant. Quo fiet, ut ipsi pauperes per civitates alienas non vagentur*' (Gaudemet and Basdevant 1989, 354-355).
[22] France, Seine-Maritime, ch.-l. cant.
[23] Bloch 1983, 57-9; Le Goff 1996, 653-57; Dulin-Aladjidi 2009, 35-57. '*Henricus rex Anglorum et dux Normannorum et Aquitanorum, et comes Andegavorum, archiepiscopis, episcopis, abbatibus, archidiaconis et omnibus ecclesie prelatis per totam terram nostram. Praecipio quatinus clericos et servientes leprosorum de Depa permittatis per parrochias*

vestras perquirere ad opus ipsorum infirmorum. Et praecipio justiciariis et ministris meis quod, si quis eis injuriam vel contumeliam fecerit, visis litteris istis, ita eis emendari et faciant ne inde eos advenire oporteat. Et finaliter prohibeo ne aliquis super eos disturbare in aliquo audeat quod ipsi infirmi et eorum hospites sunt in custodia et protectione mea' (Delisle and Berger 1916, 261 (n. 151)).
[24] '*Item apud Pontem Audomarum, quamdam domum ad opus infectorum, seu leprosorum aedificavit, qui locus vocatur sancti Aegidius: et quia ante mendicabant et victum suum quaerebant, illum locum ita fundavit, et ordonavit, ut ultra deinceps non esset illis infectis opus mendicandi nec victum suum per villam, seu patriam quaerendi: monasterium et claustrum atque dormitorium, et omnia illis necessaria, clausa et integra, ibidem aedificavit: et fratres ad servitium Dei, et dictorum infectorum, videlicet, missas et horas diei, quotidie dicentes misericorditer ordinavit*' (Du Monstier 1663, 507).
[25] France, Seine-Martime, arr. Le Havre, ch.-l. canton.
[26] '[Gautier Maloiseau] *quadam domum pauperculam leprosorum de Bolebecco aggreditur, qui de consuetudine per vicos et plateas et villas, ostiatim eleemosynas cum sabellis solebant mendicare. Qui in brevi tempore, Deo adjuvante, eos in unum retraxit eisque necessaria providit, ne ultra, pro defectu victus et vestitus, foris vagari cogerentur, sed ordinem regularem tenerent. Quatuor enim ibi ordines instituit, unum de sacerdotibus et clericis et laicis fratribus, secundum de leprosis hominibus, tertium de non sanis mulieribus, quartum de dominabus sanis et aliis famulabus*' (Arnoux 2000, 123, 300-1).
[27] Lepers are incorporated but are also being isolated: '*Leprosis autem, si fideles Christiani fuerint, Domini corporis et sanguinis participatio tribuatur; cum sanis autem convivia celebrare negentur*' (Letter of Pope Gregory II to Boniface. Dümmler 1892, 277). Rawcliffe 2006, 256.
[28] Touati 1998, 727; Rawcliffe 2006, 284-91.
[29] Gauvard 2010, 402.
[30] '*Mensura panis minorata est*' (March 17, 1248; Bonnin 1852, 34). Brown 1964, 38. '*Panem habeant ad sufficienciam, omni die. Item, soror quelibet suum vinum et suum potellum cervoisie habeat, omni die. Item, ter in hebdomada, debitis temporibus, carnes récentes habeant, et in ebdomada, semel pisces, aliis. Aliis vero diebus quinque ova, sive tria alectia, eis dentur*' (August 1249; Bonnin 1852, 101). Brown 1964, 116.
[31] Matt 14, 1-2; Mark 6, 14-16; Luke 9, 10-17; Luke 14, 12-14.
[32] Foucault 2004, 130-1.

The identity of the lepers accommodated in leper-houses was made obvious by clothing them in particular clothes akin to the monk's *habitus*. *Habitus* refers to the regulated[33] way of life depicted by Eudes Rigaud in August 1249 for the Salle-aux-Puelles.[34] The regulations he set for female lepers prescribed the use of uniform clothing covered by a russet mantle:[35]

> The raiment and clothing shall be according to that of your order and uniform, to wit, a russet mantle, and each sister shall receive a tunic and over-tunic every other year. Let them have warm mantles, and new ones every other year. Item, let the prior provide them with sufficient coverlets of fur. Item, let them have linen clothing, that is to say, two shirts and two sheets every year at least and if more are needed for those sisters who may be sick, let the prioress have them made.[36]

Edicted at almost the same time, the statutes of the Grand Beaulieu of Chartres (1264) underlined the use of a penitential colour for the clerics, and colourless for the lepers.[37] Here, the absence of colour underlined the penitential condition.[38] The rule prescribed the garment, the garment made the leper. Why were lepers made to abide by the same rules in matters of clothing as members of the clergy? Because of a common characteristic. Both clerics and lepers were separated from society by a particular ritual.

The archbishop of Rouen's visits showed the level of perceived purity the lepers had reached within the leper-houses: between the clerics and the female lepers at Mont-aux-Malades or Bellencombre,[39] healthy sisters were ranked last![40] Clothing symbolized this form of virtuous living.[41] However, the reality of such an ideal of chastity, stability and obedience remained utopian. Réginald

lived with his child. Keeping silent, one of the signs of evangelical life, was hardly enforced. Let us read the report book of the Salles-aux-Puelles:

> They mingle with the sisters and talk with them without permission. (...) Item there is over much talking in the refectory. (...) We forbade talking in the refectory or in the dormitory after Compline unless in a low voice, and briefly.[42]

The leper could but be a 'failed monk',[43] all the more so as admittance to the leper-house was not compulsory at all and did not force you into seclusion.[44] Some lepers wandered about as a result. The regulations for the Salle-aux-Puelles stipulated that part of the pittance allowed to diseased women be earmarked to feed the lepers outside.[45] Can we consider that some patients wishing to avoid the austerity inherent in leper institutions became homeless?[46] Eudes Rigaud wanted to avoid such downfall. To save the souls of the leper-women, Eudes Rigaud insisted on the need to maintain social cohesion at the Salle-aux-Puelles by obedience to the rule, a rule written down so as to guarantee brotherliness.[47] After the 1250s, the communitarian habits seemed to be no longer enforced everywhere. Whether it was at the Salle-aux-Puelles[48] or at Gournay-en-Brie,[49] meals were no longer shared despite orders to do so.

A 'priestly offensive'[50] aimed at lepers became the rule from the early 13th century, as a result of the new 'policing role' of parish priests. In 1235, the Rouen council passed most stringent laws regarding the place of lepers outside the reassuring shelter of leper-houses. It was everybody's duty to feed lepers since they had no right of citizenship.[51]

---

[33] Agamben 2011, 28-9.

[34] The leper-house was established near a deer park of Henry II at Petit-Quevilly (France, Seine-Maritime, arr. Rouen, ch.-l. canton); Grant 1994, 76-7.

[35] Davis 2006, 81.

[36] '*Vestis et habitus sint ordinati et omnibus uniformes, videlicet de rosseto, et habeat, omni anno, quelibet soror unam tunicam et supertunicale. Item, pellicias sufficientes habeant, quibuslibet duobus annis. Item, pallia sufficienta forrata, prout necessitati earum a priore videbitur expedire. Item, vestes lineas habeant, videlicet duas camisias et duo linteamina, omni anno ad minus, et si gravioribus plus oporteat fieri pro sua necessitate, fiat eis juxta arbitrium priorisse*' (January 1250; Bonnin 1852, 101-2; Brown 1964, 116-7.

[37] '1. *Habeant prior et fratres clerici capas de nigro et vestes de ronsseto clausas; habeant estivallos et non alios solutares parvos. 2. Leprosi habeant vestimenta clausa, sine colore, secundum dispositionem prioris* (Legrand 1901, 215; Pastoureau 1989, 223; Touati 1998, 413-15; Rawcliffe 2006, 303).

[38] Touati 1998, 416, 420.

[39] France, Seine-Maritime, arr. Dieppe.

[40] '*Ibi sunt quatuor conventus: unus est canonicorum, alias fratrum sanorum, tercius leprosorum, quartus leprosarum*' (January 29 1255; Bonnin 1852, 203). '*Ibi erant X canonici cum priore résidentes. Ibi erant XIX leprosi, XV leprose, XVI sorores sane*' (December 6, 1258; Bonnin 1852, 325; Brown 1964, 371. '*Ibi errant quatuor canonici cum priore, videlicet, Thomas, Guilelmus, Nicholaus et quidam senex. Item, octo leprosi, tres conversi sani, quatuor converse*' (Bellencombre, September 5, 1264; Bonnin 1852, 496; Brown 1964, 564).

[41] Agamben 2011, 86. Agamben 2012, 130-1.

[42] '*Item, verba multiplicant in refectorio* [...] *et ne loquantur cum secularibus, nisi obtenta licencia a priorissa.* [...] *Item, inhibuimus ne loquantur in refectorio et in dormitorio post completorium, nisi submissa voce et breviloquio*' (March 1248; Bonnin 1852, 34; Brown 1964, 38-39).

[43] Bériou 1991, 65.

[44] Touati 1998, 401, 405, 407, 706.

[45] '*Fragmenta vero carum pauperibus leprosis extraneis, per disposicionem prioris conserventur fideliter eroganda*' (1249; Bonnin 1852, 101; Brenner 2013, 247.

[46] Touati 1998, 682-3.

[47] '*Ob animarum salutem, duximus ordinanda, prout inferius est expressum, que ad memoriam futurorum voluimus presentibus annotari, sanctientes ipsa inviolabiliter observari*' (August 1249; Bonnin 1852, 101; Brown 1964, 116).

[48] '*Quidam clericus erat ibi leprosus, Nicholaus nomine, qui rexerat domum diutius, et comedebat frequenter in villa una cum capellano memorato, et ibidem bona domus deferabat; precipimus eidem Nicholao ne amplius se intromitteret de rebus tractantis, et capellano ne comederet cum leprosis*' (September 17, 1258; Bonnin 1852, 319; Brown 1964, 365).

[49] Seine-Maritime, Gournay-en-Bray, arr. Neufchâtel, ch.-l. cant. '*Visitamus leprosariam ejusdem loci. Ibi erant unus capellanus, quinque conversi, due converse et duo leprosi. Capellanus percipiebat ibi tantum quantum unus conversus. Inhibuimus eis ne ulterius comederent in villa, ut solebant*' (September 8, 1267; Bonnin 1852, 586; Brown 1964, 676).

[50] Vauchez 1993, 738.

[51] Touati 1998, 687. '*Ne intrent in civitates/Item inihibeant leprosis ne intrent civitatem et castella; ut dicatur eis publice in ecclesiis quod si quis injuriatus fuerit in civitate vel castello, auferendo vestes vel verberando eos, non exhibebimus eis justiciam.* [...]/8. *De iisdem, ne sedeant in tabernis/Inhibeatur etiam leprosis ne in taberna sedeant ad bibendum, etiam in villis: quia si hoc fecerint, non exhibebimus eis justiciam de injuria facta* [...]/9. *De providendo eis./Injungatur sacerdotibus ut diligenter*

If wandering lepers were not entitled to the protection of the *privilegium canonis*,[52] conversely, those lepers gathered in organised groups as defined by the 1179 council of Latran III were to be regarded as clerics, according to the *Liber pœnitentialis* (1203-13) written by Robert of Flamborough, canon of St Victor in Paris.[53] In line with him, to order a full-bodied fraternity, the 1212 Paris council and the 1214 Rouen council asked for the healthy staff of leper houses to abide by the same statute.[54]

Can we regard the 1235 ban, unenforceable anyway, as a toughening of the law, a clue to a less favourable perception of lepers, a sign of a 'change in the way lepers are looked at' which took part in the 1250-60s, as assumed by François-Olivier Touati?[55] Continuity or breakdown?

We can then understand why the ban on visiting public places occured at a time when not only the scattering of leper-houses was over and was part of the landscape,[56] but also when the amount of alms offered to leper-houses was at its peak.[57] Did the wealth of donations not deter lepers from wandering about? The Church had always prevented lepers from wandering to protect them from the mob's anger, so strong was the whiff of scandal preceding them.[58] A leper was both repellent and fascinating. Hence the need to disguise his body under garments meant to hide it from the intrusive gaze of people.

Once hidden, the taboo body of the leper was no longer the focus of attention for a crowd of people sometimes quick to adopt a violent behaviour.[59] The lepers' non sacrificial character appeared in the full covering offered by their garments, underlining their isolation from society, rigorous morals and order.[60] Comparable to the habit of a cleric who was expected to behave honourably, the 'closed' garment turned lepers into individuals whose reputation was untainted.[61] By contrast, stripping them of their garments, as anticipated in canon laws 7 and 8 of the Rouen council,[62] was akin to taking their 'status' away, to making them lose face.[63]

With no social status left, a stranger to the human community, the leper was subjected to some hostility.[64] This was all the more true as he was associated with a number of stereotypes predisposing him to join forces with the world of evil (sex, food and drink): 'a lethal troika'.[65] Béroul's *Roman de Tristan*

exemplifies this in the late 12th century.[66] How was someone's leprosy revealed? By *fama,* public rumour, neighbours, one's neighbour - in short, the crowd.[67] That slander was by essence uncontrollable.[68] In Eudes Rigaud's 1248 register, we can read that 'the priest of Hesmy[69] reported to be (*creditur*) a leper, was ill famed for incontinence'.[70] Why underline his leprosy? In towns or villages, ill *fama* contributed to defining lepers.[71] How could you get rid of this bad reputation? It seems that was the role of miracles - particularly those attributed to Thomas à Becket - to purify the leper and turn him into a new, justified being.

God's Law: overturning of the *fama*. A reading of the miracles of Thomas Becket.

The greatest figure of Anglo-Norman sainthood in the 12th century was Thomas Becket (*c.* 1120-1170). His father came from the Rouen area and his mother was a native of Caen. Thomas became Henry II's chancellor (at Christmas 1154), then was elected archbishop of Canterbury on May 21st 1162. After his assassination on December 29th 1170, the martyr's tomb became - as early as Easter 1171 - a place of popular and spontaneous worship, drawing pilgrims from places far beyond England and Normandy. A large number of miracles wrought at the shrine were recorded and documented for the canonisation trial. William of Canterbury and Benedict of Peterborough, the authors of biographies of the Saint and collections of miracles attributed to Thomas Becket, are the two main sources.[72] According to William of Canterbury, the saint was reported to have cured 34 lepers and 23 blind people, while Benedict of Peterborough only identified ten cases of leprosy, far fewer than blindness (38 cases). Out of the 367 cases of miraculous healing listed in both collections,[73] 16.62% are cases of blindness, 13.62% cases of paralysis, 11.98% cases of leprosy, while deaf and dumb people represent 2%. Twenty-two percent of the pilgrims cured of leprosy originated from Normandy. Leprosy thus stands as one of the main diseases miraculously cured in those *miracula*. Although the word *elephantiasis* tends to disappear from the 4th century onward, it was still used by Guillaume of Canterbury as synonymous with *lepra*. We have therefore counted *elephantiasis* sufferers as lepers.

The Rituals of Blood and Water

After the ban imposed on Henry II *ab ingressu ecclesiae* had been lifted by the Avranches concordat of September 27th 1172, Thomas Becket was canonised by Pope

---

moneant etiam et compellant per decanum cui hoc districte injungimus parochianos ad providendum leprosis, secundum consuetudinem talis patrie; scituri quod si super hoc audierimus questionem, eorum defectus non relinquetur impunitus' (Pontal 1983, 118-9).

[52] Génestal 1921, 40-3.
[53] Touati 1998, 403.
[54] Touati 1998, 403.
[55] Touati 1998, 685.
[56] Touati, 1998, 281-5; Jeanne 2010, 324-327.
[57] Jeanne 2010, 471.
[58] Touati 1998, 190.
[59] Gauvard 1994, 169-170; Beaune 1994, 198-99.
[60] Piponnier and Mane 1995, 164.
[61] Gauvard 2010, 393, 706.
[62] Pontal 1983, 118-9.
[63] Gauvard 2010, 706.
[64] Gauvard 2010: 523.
[65] Rawcliffe 2006, 47; Origen 1981, 25-69; Jeanne 2010, 192-195;

Gauvard 2010, 142.
[66] Touati 1998, 727; Rawcliffe 2006, 9-10.
[67] Gauvard 1994, 167-8.
[68] Gauvard 1993, 7-8; Théry 2003, 119-147.
[69] France, Seine-Maritime, commune de Preuseville, arr. Dieppe, cant. Londinières.
[70] '*Item, presbyter de Hamies, leprosus, ut creditur, infamatur est de incontinentia*' (January 19, 1248; Bonnin, 20; Brown 1964, 24.
[71] Smell of scandal was discernible before 1250-60 - see Touati 1998, 190.
[72] Benedict of Peterborough 1875; William of Canterbury 1876.
[73] Foreville 1979, 445-455.

Alexander III on February 21st, 1173. According to Guillaume of Canterbury, the secular power, in ordering Thomas' assassination, had brought down liberty, faith and charity. Thomas was shown, Christ-like, as a scapegoat, champion of the freedoms of the Church, high priest in a horsehair habit, exiled, scorned, healing the violence of a power here described as a 'leprosy' that prevented the expression of charity.

Thomas' sanctification was brought about by his martyrdom and the many miraculous healings that subsequently took place. His violent death was sublimated by the prodigies taking place around his tomb, a place of reconciliation among men. There is a kind of parallel between the violence undergone by Thomas and that borne by the leper. Both were sacred in the primitive sense. The former was cursed, assassinated, then blessed by the miracles his innocence could work. The latter, equally innocent, was also regarded as a threat to the community. The leper could only become beneficial if he had recourse to the purification operated by Thomas. The violence of the assassination and that of the disease are interchangeable since both are unclean. To proceed towards purification, the sick person has recourse to the very symbol of violence: blood, equally emblematic of Thomas' and Christ's assassinations. The documents refer to *vinage*[74] to describe a mixture of blood, water or wine drunk by sick people to purify themselves. This *vinage* copies the consecrated wine the priest drinks during the service:

> We have seen two men whose purification was perfect, and who kept no sign at all of the disease; they had received no other medicine than the water and the blood of the martyr; one of them lived near the shrine of the said martyr, eating and drinking what we had locally; his name was Richard, and he was admired by the kings, the earls, the natives, the foreigners who came to pray.[75]

The martyr's blood, like the blood of Christ shed to redeem the sinners, healed the lepers. The miraculous water renewed the water of baptism. Thus Naaman's dipping himself in Jordan seven times is a reference for the healing of leprosy and other diseases. The leper who imitated the saint who imitated Christ may hope to become clean. Pierre, a leprous monk in the monastery of St Cyprien in Poitiers, like a new Naaman, washed his wounds seven times.[76] Auger, a messenger from Robert, earl of Meulan, also washed away the leprosy of the seven deadly sins.[77]

Cleansing or Healing?

Pierre-André Sigal aptly noted that resorting to *vinage* corresponds to the dual role of medicine and religious ritual.[78] The words chosen by Benedict of Peterborough and

Guillaume of Canterbury show it well. The terminology of purification had priority over words connected to health (*sanitas*) and healing (*curo* and words derived from it).

There is a 70% occurrence of *mundo* (to clean, purge) in Benedict's volume. There too a double meaning is present. *Sanitas* refers to good health (healing) and purity. As it is, the role of the cathartic ritual is to 'mislead' violence. Cleansing lepers consisted of making them healthy again. We cannot deny that there are spontaneous cases of healing in patients suffering from tuberculoid leprosy.[79] Yet the patients do have sequels of the disease. The miracles denied the sacrificial value of the patient as a potential victim of the unleashed crowd. It worked peace among the community. The leper made clean again could no longer stand accused of all evils. The miracle expelled the idea of persecution against an exceptional being and stood for the resurrection of a doomed individual. Thanks to the saint's *præsentia*, the healed individual reintegrated into society. The miracles played a social part by cleansing someone who enjoyed no consideration from others. The pilgrimage-enforced separation from the group and the purification of the patient both contributed to violence being cured. Once healed, the patient was regarded as someone special in society, since he had benefited from a special intervention, he was chosen by God. Cleansing and healing were but one. If the collections of miracles make clear the existence of behavioural codes imposed by Benedictine monks, they also reveal people's attitudes towards leprosy. The books devoted to Thomas Becket lift a corner of the veil, allowing us to see something of what lepers had to endure in the late 12th century.

In order to arouse the reader's emotions, Becket's hagiographers promptly recorded the instances of miracles affecting the *juvenes*.[80] Leprosy, for those youths, struck in the prime of life, tragically meaning a lineage could not be continued.

Benedict of Peterborough tells the story of Gilbert, of about ten years of age, a native of Saint-Valéry-en-Caux (?) in the diocese of Rouen. This case corresponds to the rate of prevalence of the disease which reached its peak between the ages of ten and twenty[81]. The author insisted on the parents' dismay:

> Leprosy was gradually taking over the body of a young boy from Saint-Valéry, of about ten years of age, whose name was Gilbert; his hand and his arms, his feet and his legs, and all his body were in a most vicious condition. As for his face it didn't erupt in pustules but it was so swollen by a tumour with red and white spots that he was a different person altogether. Consequently, he was for his parents a great cause of pain and shame; however, having faith

[74] Sigal 2001, 35-44.
[75] William of Canterbury 1876, 332.
[76] William of Canterbury 1876, 217-9.
[77] William of Canterbury 1876, 337-8.
[78] Sigal 2001, 52.

[79] Jennekens and van Brakel 1998, 325.
[80] Duby 1978, 358.
[81] Sansarricq 1995, 55.

in God, they prayed that his sufferings might make him a cause of praise and glory.[82]

Benedict recalls the boy's metamorphosis into another being as inducing *confusio* in his parents' minds. This word is used to describe at the same time a combination of distress, shame and sadness. It indicates the combination of identities, that is to say their *loss* which causes such 'confusion'. This mimetic feeling can evolve into a sacrificial crisis characterized by a rejection of the patient. The best way to avoid such risk was to consider Gilbert as a 'martyr', offered to God in sacrifice, someone set apart ('separated'), in order to reverse the violence of the disease into widely-acknowledged glory. Losing face, losing one's identity, were the visible consequences of leprosy. By abolishing differences - you no longer knew who was who - the disease endangered the cohesion of the social body.

The religious factor tended to limit the spread of violence. Let us consider a few examples. Described as the son of a 'needy woman' (*mulieris pauperculae filius*), therefore worthless, and yet brought up in the *familia* of a rich *miles*, Richard Sunieve suffered from leprosy. He had to be evicted from his master's household and expelled from the village. His mother alone would provide for his needs:

> And God gradually spread His hand over him for eight years and He touched him, and all his body was infected with leprosy, and his flesh hurt in painful wounds. At last, as he had become a burden and a source of horror for all, merely by his being alive, he was not only kicked out of the *miles*'s household but also from the village. His mother alone accompanied him lest he perished.[83]

There was no fear of contamination in this case, but looking at the sick boy became unbearable. The feeling of repulsion that can lead to murder spread in a copycat fashion and affected all forms of community life: a knight's household, a village, a monastery. A lay brother at Boxgrove priory in Sussex begged the brothers not to make him the target of a hostile attitude while he awaited divine healing:

> For two years leprosy had been revealed on a certain Godwine, a servant of the monks of Boxgrove; he had gone seeking the heavenly physician; and until he could find Him, he begged that no weariness, no disgust, no repulsion be encouraged.[84]

How did the separation work? The system of accusation by public rumour played a major part.[85] To avoid unproven allegations, the authors of the books of miracles referred to the symptoms confirmed by tangible signs by the use of *causa* or *manifesta*.[86] Once leprosy was confirmed, the infected patients started on their pilgrimage.

The descriptions, often detailed, of the hagiographers underlined the painful reality of leprosy (a hoarse voice, nodules), enabling them to extol the virtues of the saint, dispenser of purity. Without yielding to a sorrowful vision of the *miracula*, one cannot help wondering about the patients' individual reactions. Admittedly, the disease traced an ideal path towards penitence, and the monks endlessly repeated the words from the Epistle of Paul to the Hebrews (12, 6) that says God chastens those he loves. Despite the yearning for redemption that dominated the ecclesiastical speech, the reality of the disease remained hard to accept. In what way did this (relative) separation of the lepers constitute - rather paradoxically - a process of union?

Lepers could see their diseased life as an injustice. In that case, they regarded themselves as victims. The Church reminded them of Job's example.[87] Sometimes, the disease was perceived as the consequence of an individual or collective transgression of the social rules, demanding some form of atonement, a 'socializing action',[88] that is to say a repentance which corresponded, according to the clerics' norms, to admission into the leper-house. The offence vanished and social order was preserved: the patient ran no more risks. He did not become a 'freak' and could no longer be the victim of the mob's opprobrium.

Guillaume of Canterbury gave the example of Jean, a priest and a leper saved by Thomas Becket:

> John, a priest whose evidence can be trusted, left the place of Nottingham to honour the memory of Thomas the martyr. He left on account of the leprosy that caused him to be misshapen and made him worthless (horrible). Back home after three days, his condition worsened, with dreadful, bulging pustules, facial hair getting scarce, and his face deteriorating so badly that he could not partake of the common society. This is why he was reduced to leaving his lodgings for the company of the co-leper brothers; having passed an agreement with them, he cohabited with them.[89]

The priest was forced to leave Nottingham because the leprosy he contracted had made him the butt of the population's scorn. After three days, he was in such a state that he literally lost face. Now beardless, he found his manliness gone. He was then taken inside the leper community. Arrival among the 'leprous companions' conveyed, with the use of the verb *sordere*, the protection of a 'worthless' individual. It was now impossible for him to live within a society that rejected him. He changed norms and would from then on share the life of a group of people suffering from the same disease.

---

[82] William of Canterbury 1875, 244-5.
[83] William of Canterbury 1875, 246.
[84] William of Canterbury 1876, 339.
[85] Girard 1991, 25, 81.
[86] William of Canterbury 1876, 222, 293, 330, 429.

[87] Touati 1998, 198.
[88] Brown 1984, 155.
[89] William of Canterbury 1875, 330.

In a letter written *c.* 1174 supporting Thomas A Becket's canonisation, Stephen (*c.* 1159-89), prior of the Augustinian House of Saint Peter and Saint Paul in Taunton,[90] removed John the King - a canon affected by leprosy - from the community:

> Thus, by the judgement of God, he was smitten by a serious and manifest form of leprosy. From that moment, we were afraid of the danger of that disease and set him apart from the community of our brethren, we entrusted his care to a poorhouse in the vicinity of our church, supplying all the necessaries for his well-being. [...] A particular John nicknamed The King, started wasting away, losing his hair and his beard, and being deformed by tumours; he lived yet another two years in the Taunton house, our brothers partaking of his suffering as much as his disabilities made it possible. But as the disease carries the evil eye to the co-habitants, he was removed to a hospice for patients suffering from the same evil.[91]

In the early stages of his disease, he had been regarded compassionately by the canonical brotherhood, but that attitude did not last. For what reason? Because canon John's leprosy was threatening the brothers' cohesion. In order to understand this sudden change of attitude, the keyword is *invidire*. It means precisely: cast malevolent, evil looks, cast the evil eye, act malevolently, want to spite. Removing John did not proceed from precautions against a contagious disease, but from the fear of the group's loss of cohesion.

The canons' attitude fluctuated from care to rejection. The latter prevailed. John was set apart from the community for his medical condition to be adequately treated but also to protect him from the suspicion of casting the evil eye on the other canons.[92] If leprosy is evil-bearing, then the leper is victimised. Next came the accusation of undermining the cohesion of the group as the leper benefited from a different treatment justified by his disease. Accepted initially as a divine *signum*, the disease quickly turned into a burden. The way of life of the sick man did not conform any more with the Augustinian rule's expected behaviour: John was no longer acknowledged as one of them by the brotherhood of canons. He had to leave. This too often overlooked aspect is very important to understand one of the factors triggering the eviction, yet prevents us from

understanding why, in accordance with the dual logic of care-giving and setting the lepers aside.[93] The leper was suspected of threatening the Taunton community and therefore had to be removed.

That brand of scandal marking the leper is not peculiar to the 12th century. It is to be found again a century later, in the book in which Rouen archbishop Eudes Rigaud kept a record of his pastoral visits. On April 3rd 1269, Eudes Rigaud paid a visit to the Benedictine abbey of Bec Hellouin. He remarked that one of the brothers, Nicholas of Lendy, was suspected of leprosy (*suspectus de lepra*). That monk aroused general abomination. It was a tricky situation. Here was a monastery of 43 monks and 20 novices,[94] all seeming to unite against one! We don't know whether Nicholas of Lendy's future was debated in chapter. After he had consulted with the archbishop in the privacy of the cell where he usually slept on his visits, the abbot decided to send him to the leper-house of Saint-Lambert, attached to Bec Hellouin since the 12th century.[95] The private interview made it possible to settle a scandal, that of the monks' violence, as well as Nicholas' inability to fulfil his duties:

Item, since the community [of Bec] suspected Brother Nicholas of Lendy of leprosy, and abhorred and abominated him because of this, we advised the abbot privately, in the chamber where we, as of custom, slept, to send the said Brother Nicholas away. The abbot told us that he would send him to St-Lambert's, where there is no great concourse of men and where he might receive the benefit of the air and considerable mitigation of his ailment.[96]

The main function of the rite of entry into the leper-house was to avoid a return to the sacrificial crisis. Its role was to prevent rather than cure violence. This sublimation of the victims that offered themselves founded a new community. It was a rite of entry that can be compared to a *profession*:[97] it was a sacrificial offering of oneself, the aim of which was to drive violence away.

Bonding together in leper communities: setting apart in order to unite

Some American biologists have recently come up with the theory of a possible correlation between the recurring presence of epidemics of infectious diseases and the apparition of religions as factors of mutual assistance and collective grouping;[98] this theory calls for a re-evaluation

---

[90] Somersetshire, England, diocese of Wells. Priory of Saint Augustine founded *c.* 1115.

[91] '*Divino ita procurante judicio lepra gravi et manifesta fuisse percussum. Unde et nos, hujusmodi infirmitatis timentes periculum eum a coetu fratrum nostrorum segregatum ad quandam domum pauperum, ecclesie nostrae conterminam, providentes ei vitae necessaria delegavimus*'. [...] '*Qui Johannes nominatus et Rex cognominatus, cum capillis et barba defluentibus deflorari et deformari tuberibus inciperet, adhuc in domo Tantonensi per biennum resedit, fratri fratribus quantum permitteret infirmitas compatientibus. Sed cohabitationi cum morbus invideret, in xenodochium simili morbo laborantium segregatus est*' (William of Canterbury 1875, 429-30).

[92] An element overlooked by Carol Rawcliffe, who considers that John's physical condition is the sole factor leading to his being moved to a leper-house (Rawcliffe 2006, 172).

[93] Girard 2002a, 40-1.

[94] '*Invenimus ibi LXIIII monachos* [...] *viginti de dictis sexaginta quatuor errant novicii*' (Bonnin 1852, 623; Brown 1964, 716).

[95] Baudot 1993, 107-9.

[96] '*Item, quia conventus habebat fratrem Nicholaum de Lendy suspectus de lepra, et abborreat eum propter hoc et abhominatur, consuluimus abbati secreto, in camera ubi consuevimus jacere, quod dictum fratrem N. ab inde amoveret; et dixit nobis quod ipsum ad locum Sancti-Lamberti mitteret, ubi non est frequentia hominum, ubique beneficium aeris et multa infirmitatis sue levamenta habere posset*' (Bonnin 1852, 623; Brown 1964, 717).

[97] Touati 1998, 399-402; Kupfer 2003, 143; Rawcliffe 2006, 20; 302-3.

[98] Fincher and Thornhill 2008, 2587-2594; Fincher, Thornhill *et al* 2008,

of the place and role of disease-related religious attitudes. Anthropologically, Claude Lévi-Strauss had, as early as 1949, established a link between multi-shaped crises and spontaneous social aggregations, yet he did not see in them a parallel rise in religious phenomena.[99].

The phenomenon of lepers spontaneously getting together pre-dated the institution: words first described the lepers (*leprosi*) and then the leper house (*domus leprosorum*),[100] the founding of which could result from their being stigmatized, as observed for instance in *Ami and Amile,*[101] (*c.* 1200), which would validate Claude Lévi-Strauss' and the American biologists' theory. Even in the 12th century, the game of medieval alms-giving never emanated from a 'kind-hearted and benevolent' *caritas.*[102] It was a ritual oscillating from scorn to pity.[103] Thus we would see the constitution of evangelical associations of assistance to the lepers akin to the French confraternities Catherine Vincent has reviewed.[104] The 1179 third Lateran council ensured the stability of those brotherhoods by directing that they be run by a priest and set up in a particular hospice, together with its own church and graveyard. When you were identified as a leper, you were granted the right to physical and spiritual care in a leper house. How did you come by that identification as a leper?

The only leper entity to be acknowledged was collective. It followed an *ordo* defined by rigorous terminology;[105] the words referring to the leper-communities in the 12th century bear the monastic stamp. Bois Halbout's lepers around 1160 referred to themselves as *humiles servi Deo.*[106] As for the Bayeux leper community, it was self-described as a monastery.[107]

A leper's admittance ritual ceremony was similar to that of a layman in mortal danger being admitted to a monastery.[108] As early as in the 10th century, in the monastic infirmaries, people about to die could be received into the community according to *ad succurendum* rites.[109] Spurred on by the Bec Hellouin 'school' in the early 12th century,[110] that rite could be interpreted as a double separation preceeding a double union: severance from one's family to join a

monastic brotherhood; refusal of death to join the just in eternal life. Such practice can be observed in a late 12th century charter noted down in the cartulary of St Stephen's Abbey in Caen, which counted St Thomas' leper-house among its properties.[111]

Joining a leper-house was made possible through a ritual of self-renunciation (which became visible with the adoption of the monastic habit) and oath-taking, as can be seen for instance in Saint-Lazarus of Montpellier circa 1150 or in Saint-Lazarus of Noyon a century later.[112] Was swearing obedience to the monastic rule the same as cutting oneself off from society to produce a union, that of the lepers' brotherhood?[113] Or is the ritual a case of degrading the leper, aiming at speeding up his death, as John Bossy suggests?[114] It seems that the admittance ceremony was double-edged, with a negative and a positive side. Death to the world presented the dark side of the ritual: it validated a separation. The light side stood for membership of a leper brotherhood. On what model was that ritual patterned? The leper could be apprehended as a 'christomimetic'[115] suffering *hostia* (victim), referring to the image of St Hieronymus '*Christus quasi leprosus*',[116] an image used again by Gerbert, abbot of St-Wandrille (1063-89).[117]

The ceremony could be assimilated with the breaking of the host during mass. Christ is torn, denuded and broken.[118] The leper is also similarly stripped. The first rite stood for the sacrificial death of the historic Christ,[119] the second lay the foundations of a public conversion evolving into a blood-free sacrifice symbolically reiterating the sacrifice of Christ consecrated once and for all.[120] In my opinion, there is no need to call on the studies of Zambia's Ndembu by Victor Turner[121] since all medieval ceremonies are based

1279-2585.

[99] Lévi-Strauss 1969, 42, 60.

[100] Touati 1998, 266, 399-400.

[101] '*Fiz a mezel, a delgiet et a ladre! / Ja n'iert uns jors que por lui ne voz bate*' Dembrowski 1969, 72.

[102] Roch 1989, 505-06, 508, 510.

[103] '*Li uns, ausi que par courous, / Li dist: "Truans, fuiés, fuiés / Batus u en la mer plonciés / Serés ancui, s'on me veut croire, / Au paiement de ceste foire*' Wilmotte 1927, 19.

[104] Vincent 1994, 70-73.

[105] Legrand 1901, VII.

[106] Arnoux and Maneuvrier 2001, 48 (n. 26c).

[107] '*Confirmasse in perpetum ellemosinam XX prebendas quas Willemus illustris Rex Anglorum, per avus meus stabilivit de redditibus suis in civitate Baiocas, confratribus leprosis in monasterio Sancti Nicholai Baiocas sub religione viventibus sunt*' Library of Bayeux, ms 1 cartulary of St. Nicolas: f. 1 (n. 1).

[108] Touati 1991, 8-9, 17-18; Touati 1998; 39, 46-47; Jeanne 1997, 573-592.

[109] De Miramon 1999, 123.

[110] Grandjean 1994, 247; De Miramon 1999, 49; Leclercq 1955, 158-168; Gougaud 1925, 129-142. To compare: Lefèvre 1932, 289-307.

[111] '*Guillelmus Rufus et duo filii ejus primogeniti dederunt nobis et posuerunt super altare beati Stephani VI acras terre in territorio de Fontibus et de Stupefor super viam juxta crucem acram et dimidiam in Longis Boellis, III acras in duabus peciis ad Longam reiam dimidiam acram super viam de Baron, I acram dimidiam virgata unius. Nos autem recepimus Barthum fratrem predicti Willelmi qui erat leprosus in domo leprosorum nostrorum in burgo nostro et usque ad finem vite sue ei victui necessaria invenimus*' (End of 12th century - Caen, Arch. dép. Calvados, 1J41 Cartulary of St. Stephen of Caen, f 88v, 270).

[112] '*Hec sunt precepta que salutem animarum suarum eis subsecuntur: si misellus vel misella, leprosus vel leprosa recepi in domo voluerit, primum se Deo dare et servire, et hobedienciam aministratoribus promittat. Si dixerit se nullam velle promittere obedienciam, non recipiatur*'. [...] '*Item que ledit frère ou sereur renonche à ladicte maison l'an ou fache profecion et regidence, se che n'est par le congié du maistre, des frères et des sereurs. Item, que les frères ayent l'habit...*' Legrand 1901, 182, 195.

[113] Jacob 2006, 581; Bickerman 1976, 1-32; Scubla 1998, 56; Tarot 2012, 263-292.

[114] Bossy 1983, 46; Moore 2007, 57.

[115] Kantorowicz 1997, 47, 48, 49, 58,143.

[116] '*Vere languores nostros ipse tulit et dolores nostros portavit. Et nos putavimus eum quasi leprosum et percussum a Deo, et humiliatum*' (Adriaen 1963, 587-9).

[117] '*Speciosus ille in gloria Jesus, quasi leprosus portans nostri languoris ulcera et suo livore sanans nos in crucis dolore, ut fas et dignum est, crucifixus gloriatur per orbem, dignus corde, dignus calamo scribae, dignus pincello picturae, litteratis et idiotis ad lectionem dibitae recordationis*' (Dolbeau 2002, 227).

[118] Bossy 1983, 49.

[119] Hocart 1927, 157-61; Hocart 1954, 82.

[120] Bossy 1983, 50-51, 53; Heb. 10, 9.

[121] Rawcliffe 2006, 42.

Christ's passion	A king's coronation	A monk's profession of faith	Isolation of a leper
Jesus is arrested by the Romans	'kidnapping' of 'sleeping king' by the bishops of Beauvais and Laon	Abbot and monastic community fetch the novice	The priest and the crowd go and fetch the sick man
Jeers, flogging, parody of a coronation	One of them utters a prayer asking the king to share salvation among all	Abbot exhorts novice to patience and foretells a martyr's life	The priest exhorts the leper to patience and gives him his blessing
On his way to Golgotha (skull) Insults	Procession to cathedral. Crucifix ahead of procession. Acclamations from the crowd	Procession to the oratory crucifix ahead of procession	Procession to the church crucifix ahead of procession
Jesus sheds his clothes, divided among the soldiers	Oath *Te Deum* The king stands before the altar and removes the upper layer of his former clothes	Vow of poverty *Petitio* placed on altar	The leper vows to renounce worldly goods *Donatio* placed on altar
Crucifixion The thieves jeer at Jesus Jesus dies	Dubbing The king lies on floor, with stretched arms (or kneels with head bent) while clerics around him chant litanies Anointment	Monk kneels, head bent while monastic community around him chants litanies	The leper kneels under a catafalque to hear mass Confession Tonsure (sometimes) Enactment of burial
Resurrection Christ-King Death to the world and rebirth	*Insignia* given to him, the king is dressed in coronation robes. He is crowned by Rheims archbishop. He ascends to the X-shaped (chrism) throne Mass. Like a priest, king takes holy communion (wine and bread). The king is blessed and shows himself to the people Procession from cathedral to palace	The monk is tonsured and puts on the cloister's habits Abbot reads the rule	Procession to leper-house Blessed by the priest, the leper is welcomed and dressed in a frock, in leper-house or outside his hut ('borde' in french) 'defences' read out to prevent the patient from arousing contagious violence among the crowd

TABLE 1. 'UNITY OF ALL RITES': THE CEREMONIAL OF DEATH AND REBIRTH

on the remembrance of Christ's sacrifice. As in the case of a king's anointment, a knight's accolade, or a monk's profession, one phase of the leper's admittance ritual involved a vesting ceremony symbolizing passage from one condition to another: sinner to penitent (Table 1).[122] It is a fact that written descriptions only occur towards the late 15th century, but François-Olivier Touati regarded it as a deep-rooted practice fossilized by the printed word.[123]

Because the ritual unfolded in the manner of a funeral, it struck people's imagination and gave way to many more or less sensational descriptions. Françoise Bériac once classified the separation *ordines* without realizing they were variations on a unique ritual that did not need to be written down in order to exist.[124] Strictly oral transmission is a better preserver of the fundamental patterns, yet it admits faster variations of detail.[125] It therefore allows for an abundance of details within a rigid framework.

Why did the liturgical codification of the lepers appear so late? We may consider several factors. Catherine Vincent studied Rouen and Paris obituaries and observed that lay

[122] Touati 1998, 411.
[123] Touati 1998, 410-412.

[124] Bériac 1985, 253-55.
[125] Chaunu 2003, 167.

people were asking for more and more demanding funeral services after 1450. That movement took place later than in the South and was not linked to the spreading of the Purgatory liturgy - the accumulation of elections had more to do with the communion of saints - but related more to the worry of a second death plunging the faithful in oblivion.[126] That anguish before oblivion is to be connected with what Pierre Chaunu called 'the time of collective death' (1348-75) of the plague epidemics, which would incite the faithful to manifest clearer penitential attitudes.[127]

The rite of segregation of the lepers - which was performed out of habit and whose significance had been lost - took on a new meaning with the plague. With the growth of the notion of 'contagion' after 1350, the lepers' segregation ceremony was interpreted as an answer to that new data. From then on, the old 13th century segregation of lepers and what they were forbidden[128] could be seen as a reference to be used for all patients suspected of carrying the disease. One can understand why lepers were the butt of the renewal of old stereotypes.[129]

Another sign of distrust towards those lepers whose disease was so frightening was the fine imposed on the brothers if they did not abide by the rites. The fine was small, not more than a few *deniers*. Its amount was not what mattered however, but the dishonour incurred if the norm was not respected.[130] These fines appeared rather late, the first known was codified in the statute-book of Caen's St Sauveur in 1480.[131]

René Girard underlined the idea that there is nothing irrational in the perception that a great plague epidemic was likely to bring about a social collapse.[132] Jacques Despars, a physician (†1458) was quite right when he insisted on the harm caused by fear in his comments on Avicenne's *Canon*.[133] Denise Angers pointed out that between 1396 and 1500, the public notarial books of Caen recorded more and more dramatized obituaries, with specific requests for prayers, hymns, processions, and a chosen burial site.[134]

In Normandy, charities gathered brothers united in their reverence in the face of death.[135] Who indeed could outdo the charities in their concern about the fate of those of their brothers who had become 'dead to the world' on being affected by leprosy? We may wonder to what extent these praying fraternities may have been one of the repositories of the rite of segregation of lepers. When the statutes were written down in the 1440s, clerks systematically mention the procession leading to the leper-house or to the 'usual place'.[136] A procession was illustrated in *Ami and Amile*.[137] Catherine Vincent rightfully points out that two cases of help are connected to members regarded as 'dead' by the association, and getting, as such, a service akin to a funeral service: pilgrim brothers and leper brothers.[138]

Promoting such rites also seems to fit in the *devotio moderna* movement, '*imitatio Christi*' of the God of sufferings turned Man, similar to the leper. Its impact in Normandy ought to be measured however. *Devotio moderna* is an individual recourse[139] which could fit in well with the loss of community life in leper-houses.

The purpose of these rites was to allow for a (relative) banishment of the leper, who until then was the carrier of the impure sacredness (*sacer*), but was turned into clean sacredness (*sanctus*).

By joining his peers in a praying community, he became useful for society, being used as a model of life; in England, at Dover's leper-house, the lepers were tonsured like monks.[140] The establishment of leper-houses derived from this rite and not the reverse. We think this is confirmed by the existence of leper-communities before their institution.[141]

The rite does indeed come before the institution: by joining a leper-community, you will imitate Christ in a life of repentance. Joining such a community also meant you became stronger, for anyone becoming ill and isolated, without the support of one's family, one's church, one's master, or penniless, becomes *debilis* or *pauper*. The leper brotherhood was not imposed from above, but like all communities, arose from a need.[142] By settling in a particular place under the protection of God and the saints, the lepers not only found salvation, but also the assurance of food and adequate care, and a peaceful death.

So the lepers reorganized their lives according to their disability. They joined forces together in groups of the same eschatological category, judging by the vocabulary used by the clerics, borrowed from the evangelical ideal of the 1170s of '*fratres colleprosos*'.[143] To achieve

---

[126] Vincent 1991, 137-149.

[127] Chaunu 2003, 186; 194.

[128] Status of leper-house of Lisieux (1256):'*Noverint universitas vestra q[ui] aliquis leprosorum dicte leprosarie non debet, nec potest transire doitum de Tou[qu]a sine licencia et jussu presbiteri vel alius a dicto presbitero deputati*' (Legrand 1901, 203).

[129] Touati 1998, 727.

[130] Jeanne 2012, 189-202.

[131] '*Item, s'il advient qu'aucun des dits frères ou sœurs échisse en maladie de mesellerie ou autre par quoy il fust séparé de la compagnie humaine, et il requiert avoir des biens d'icelle charité, on luy en aidera jusques a la somme de vingt sols tournois, et aura une basse messe en la paroisse dont il partira ou lieu dessus dit de Saint-Sauveur et sera convoyé des dits jusques au lieu acoustumé, sur peine de l'amende dessus dite [deux deniers selon l'art. III du statut]*' (Caen, Arch. dép. Calvados, G 1020).

[132] Girard 2002b, 229.

[133] Jacquart 1998, 257.

[134] Regretfully, there is not much emphasis on the chronological evolution of practices, based on data contained in over a hundred deeds: Angers 2010, 18.

[135] Chaunu 2003, 198.

[136] The first statute to be drafted is that of the Saint Eustache brotherhood in the church of Notre-Dame de Froide rue in Caen: Caen, Arch. dép. Calvados: G 887.

[137] '*Lubias prinst un ostel qui fu viéz / Par defors Balivies, la le fist harbagier. / Procession i fait grant li clergier, / Puis s'en retornent en la cité arriers. Dex com grant duel demainnent!*' (Dembrowski 1969, 71).

[138] Vincent 1988, 42, 31, 146-7, 164.

[139] Chaunu 2003, 259-60, 356.

[140] Rawcliffe 2006, 303.

[141] Bériac 1990, 18.

[142] Vincent 1994, 31; 47.

[143] William of Canterbury 1875, 330.

salvation, these 'brothers' submitted to a monastic-like religious rule, in a place of mutual help, organized around prayer and divine worship: the '*domus leprosorum*', the '*monasterium*' or the '*conventus leprosorum*'.[144] '*Leprosaria*' or '*maladeria*' are very seldom used.

Conclusion

As early as the 6th century, begging by lepers was condemned as a source of unrest. In the 13th century, laws banning leper vagrancy were reiterated and toughened, at a time when it was deemed there were sufficient numbers of leper houses in France. From then on, statutory lepers were sick people entering the leper house in a public and official ceremony and putting on the penitent's garb. They lived together as a group submitting to a rule and were the only beneficiaries of public almsgiving. They were honourable since their *habitus* made their life closer to that of a monk than of a poor wretch (*mésel*) begging for bread and rousing the passers-by's animosity.

Study of the books recording the miracles attributed to Thomas Becket and the pastoral visits of Eudes Rigaud shows that the life of lepers in a monastery or a canon's community disturbed the order of the *Opus Dei*. As a result, in order to escape the animosity of their fellow-brothers, they had to leave the community and join a leper-brotherhood. Attracting a saint's favour by taking part in a pilgrimage enabled them to acquire a new identity in order to be accepted by all. By contrast, wandering lepers had no identity; they were non-justiciable outsiders whose fate became precarious in the days of the recurring plague epidemics of the 14th and 15th centuries. They had lost face.

---

[144] '*Confratribus leprosis in monasterio Sancti-Nicholai Baiocas sub religione viventibus sunt*'; '*Sancti-Nicholai Baiocensis leprosorum conventus*' Library of Bayeux, ms 1 cartulary of Saint-Nicolas, f. 1, n. 2 (c. 1170); f. 16, n. 19 (c. 1215-33).

Bibliography

Adriaen, M. (ed.) 1963. *S. Hieronymi presbyteri commentariorum in Esaiam libri XII-XVIII in Esaia parvula adbrevatio,* Turnhout: Brepols.

Agamben, G. (trans. Gayraud, J.) 2011. *De la très haute pauvreté. Règles et formes de vie (Homo sacer, IV, 1),* Paris: Bibliothèque Rivages et Payot.

Agamben, G. 2012. *Opus Dei. Archéologie de l'office. (Homo Sacer, II, 5),* Paris: Le Seuil.

Angers, D. 2010. '"Meu en devocion, et pensant au prouffit et salut de l'ame de lui et de tous ses parens..." Les bourgeois de Caen, la mémoire et l'au-delà (1396-1500)', *Tabularia 'Études',* **10,** 1-39.

Arnoux, M. 2000. *Des clercs au service de la réforme. Études et documents sur les chanoines réguliers dans la province de Rouen,* Turnhout: Brepols.

Arnoux, M. and Maneuvrier, C. 2001. *Deux abbayes de Basse-Normandie: Notre-Dame du Val et le Val Richer (XIIe–XIIIe siècles),* Flers: Le Pays Bas-Normand, **1-2** (237-238).

Baudot, M. 1993. 'Un prieuré de l'abbaye du Bec-Hellouin dans la tourmente de la guerre de Cent Ans? Le prieuré de Saint-Lambert à Fontaine-la-Soret', *Annales de Normandie,* **2,** 107-23.

Beaune, C. 1994. 'La rumeur dans le *Journal du Bourgeois de Paris',* in *La circulation des nouvelles au Moyen Âge,* 191-203. Paris and Rome: Publications de la Sorbonne.

Bériac, F. 1985. 'Mourir au monde. Les *ordines* de séparation des lépreux en France aux XVe et XVIe siècles', *Journal of medieval history,* **11,** 253-55.

Bériou, N. 1991. 'Les lépreux sous le regard des prédicateurs d'après les collections des sermons *Ad status* du XIIIe siècle', in N. Bériou and F.O. Touati (eds), *Voluntate Dei leprosus. Les lépreux entre conversion et exclusion aux XIIe et XIIIe siècles,* 33-80. Spoleto: Fondazione CISAM.

Bickerman, É. 1976. 'Couper une alliance', in *Studies in Jewish and Christian History,* 1: 1-32. Leiden: Brill.

Bloch, M. 1983. *Les rois thaumaturges. Étude sur le caractère surnaturel attribué à la puissance royale particulièrement en France et en Angleterre,* Paris: Gallimard.

Bonnin, T. (ed.) 1852. *Regestrum visitationum archiepiscopi Rothomagensis: Journal des visites pastorales d'Eudes Rigaud, archevêque de Rouen, MCCXLVIII-MCCLXIX,* Rouen: A. Le Brument.

Borret, M. (ed), 1981. *Origen: Homélies sur le Lévitique,* 2 Vols, Paris: Le Cerf.

Bossy, J. 1983. 'The mass as a social institution 1200-1700', *Past and Present* **100(1),** 29-61.

Brenner, E. 2013. 'The leprous body in twelfth and thirteenth century Rouen: perceptions and responses', in S. Conklin Akbari and J. Ross (eds), *The Ends of the Body. Identity and Community in Medieval Culture,* 239-259. Toronto: Toronto University Press.

Brown, P. (2007), Le culte des saints: Son essor et sa fonction dans la chrêtienté latine, Paris: Les Éditions du Cerf.

Brown, S.M. (ed.) 1964. *The register of Eudes of Rouen,* New York: Columbia University Press.

Cartulary of the leper-house of St. Nicolas of Bayeux, Bayeux: Médiathèque municipale: Ms 1

Cartulary of St. Stephen of Caen, Caen: Archives départementales du Calvados: 1J41 G 887; G 1020.

Chaunu, P. 2003. *Le temps des Réformes. Histoire religieuse et système de civilisation. La crise de la chrétienté. L'Éclatement (1250-1550),* Paris: Hachette.

Dalarun, J. 2012. *Gouverner, c'est servir. Essai de démocratie médiévale,* Paris: Alma.

Davis, A.J. 2006. *The Holy Bureaucrat. Eudes Rigaud and Religious Reform in Thirteenth-Century Normandy,* Ithaca: Cornell University Press.

Delisle, L. and Berger, E. (eds) 1916. *Recueil des Actes de Henri II (3 Vols).* Paris: Imprimerie Nationale

Demaitre, L. 2007. *Leprosy in Premodern Medicine: A Malady of the Whole Body,* Baltimore: The Johns Hopkins University Press.

Dembrowski, P.F. (ed.), 1969. *Ami et Amile. Chanson de geste,* Paris: Honore Champion.

Dolbeau, F. 2002. 'Passion et résurrection du Christ, selon Gerbert, abbé de Saint-Wandrille († 1089)', *Latin Culture in the Eleventh Century, The Journal of Medieval Latin,* **5(1),** 223-249.

Duby, G. 1978. *Les trois ordres ou l'imaginaire du féodalisme,* Paris: Gallimard.

Dulin-Aladjidi, P. 2009. *Le Roi père des pauvres. France, XIIIe–XVe siècle,* Rennes: Presses Universitaires de Rennes.

Dümmler, E. (ed.) 1892. *Monumenta Germaniae Historica, Epistolae Merovingici et Karolini Aevi I,* letter 26, Berlin: Weidmann.

Du Monstier, A. (ed.) 1663. *Neustria pia seu de omnibus et singulis abbatiis et prioratibus totius Normaniae,* Rouen.

Durkheim, É. 1912 (repr. 2008). *Les Formes élémentaires de la vie religieuse. Le système totémique en Australie,* Paris: Presses Universitaires de France.

Fincher C.L., Thornhill, R., Murray, R.D.R. and Schaller, M. 2008. 'Pathogen prevalence predicts human cross-cultural variability in individualism/collectivism', *Proceedings of the Royal Society,* **275,** 1279-2585.

Fincher C.L. and Thornhill, R. 2008. 'Assortive sociability, limited dispersal, infectious disease and the genesis of the global pattern of religion diversity', *Proceedings of the Royal Society,* **275,** 2587-2594.

Foreville, R. 1979. 'Les "Miracula /s. Thomae Cantuarensis"', *ACNSS, 97 (1972); Section de Philologie et d'Histoire jusqu'a 1610,* 443-68. Paris: Bibliotheque Nationale.

Foucault, M. 2004. *Sécurité, territoire, population. Cours au Collège de France, 1977-1978,* Paris: Gallimard.

Foucault, M. 2012. *Du gouvernement des vivants. Cours au collège de France (1979-1980),* Paris: Gallimard.

Gaudemet, J. and Basdevant, B. (eds) 1989. *Canons des conciles mérovingiens (VIe-VIIe siècles)* Vol. 1, Paris: Le Cerf.

Gauvard, C. 1993. 'La *fama*, une parole fondatrice', *Médiévales*, **24**, 5-13.

Gauvard, C. 1994. 'Rumeurs et stéréotypes à la fin du Moyen Âge', in *La circulation des nouvelles au Moyen Âge*, 157-177. Paris and Rome: Publications de la Sorbonne.

Gauvard, C. 2010. *'De grace especial'. Crime, État et société en France à la fin du Moyen Âge*, Paris: Publications de la Sorbonne.

Génestal, R. 1921. *Le privilegium fori en France du décret de Gratien au XIVe siècle* (2 vols), Paris: Éditions Ernest Leroux.

Girard, R. 1991. *Le Bouc émissaire*, Paris: Librairie générale française

Girard, R. 2002a. 'Violence et représentation dans le texte mythique', in *La voix méconnue du réel. Une théorie des mythes archaïques et modernes*, 27-63. Paris: Grasset.

Girard, R. 2002b. 'La peste dans la littérature et le mythe' in *La voix méconnue du réel. Une théorie des mythes archaïques et modernes*: 227-261. Paris: Grasset.

Girard, R. 2006. *La violence et le sacré*, Paris: Librairie générale française.

Gougaud, L. 1925. 'Mourir sous le froc', in *Dévotions et pratiques ascétiques au Moyen Âge*: 129-142. Paris: Descleé de Brouwe 2.

Grandjean, M. 1994. *Laïcs dans l'Église. Regards de Pierre Damien, Anselme de Cantorbéry, Yves de Chartres*, Paris: Beauchesne.

Grant, L. 1994. 'Le patronage architectural d'Henri II et de son entourage', *Cahiers de Civilisation médiévale*, **38**, 73-84.

Hocart, A.M. 1927. *Kingship*, Oxford: Oxford University Press.

Hocart, A.M. 1954. *Social Origins*, London: Watts.

Huizinga, J. 1924 (repr. 1987). *The Waning of the Middle Ages: a Study of the Forms of life, Thought, and Art in France and the Netherlands in the Fourteenth and Fifteenth centuries*, London: Penguin Books.

Jacob, R. 2006. 'La question romaine du *sacer*. Ambivalence du sacré ou construction symbolique de la sortie du droit', *Revue historique*, **639(3)**, 523-88.

Jacquart, D. 1998. *La médecine médiévale dans le cadre parisien, XIVe–XVe siècle*, Paris: Fayard.

Jeanne, D. 1997. 'Des évêques et des lépreux. Essai sur la pastorale de séparation du lépreux dans la province ecclésiastique de Rouen à partir des synodes et des rituels diocésains, XVe-XVIIe siècles', in S. Lemagnen and P. Manneville (eds), *Cathédrales et chapitres en Normandie*, 573-592. Caen: Musée de Normandie.

Jeanne, D. 2012. '"Condempné et desclaré estre ladre": Simon Lecourt un"'riche marchant tanneur" qui perd la face: essai d'anthropologie historique sur le bouc émissaire', in M. Hamon and A. Rovere (eds), *Être reconnu de son temps: personnalité et notables aux Temps modernes*, 189-202. Édition électronique du CTHS.

Jeanne, D. 2010. *Garder ou perdre la face? La Maladie et le Sacré. Étude d'anthropologie historique sur la lèpre (Normandie centrale, occidentale et méridionale) du XIe au XVIe siècle*, Thèse d'histoire nouveau régime, Université Paris-Ouest-Nanterre-la-Défense, 3 vols.

Jennekens, F.G.I. and van Brakel, W.H. 1998. 'Neuropathy in leprosy', in N. Latov, J.H.J Wokke, and J.J. Kelly (eds), *Immunological and Infectious Diseases of the Peripheral Nerves*, 319-339. Cambridge: CUP.

Kantorowicz, E. 1997. *The King's Two Bodies: a Study in Medieval Political Theology*, Princeton: Princeton University Press.

Kupfer, M. 2003. *The Art of Healing: Painting for the Sick and the Sinner in a Medieval Town*, University Park: Pennsylvania State University Press.

Le Blévec, D. 2000. *La part du pauvre. L'assistance dans les pays du Bas-Rhône du XIIe au milieu du XVe siècle* (2 vols.), Rome: École Française de Rome.

Leclercq, J. 1955. 'La vêture *ad succurendum* d'après le moine Raoul', *Analecta monastica. Textes et études sur la vie des moines au Moyen Âge*, **37(3)**, 158-168.

Lefèvre, P. 1932. 'Les cérémonies de la vêture et de la profession dans l'ordre de prémontré', *Analecta Præmonstratensia*, **8**, 289-307.

Legrand, L. (ed.) 1901. *Statuts d'hôtels-Dieu et de léproseries. Recueils de textes du XIIe au XIVe siècle*, Paris: Picard.

Le Goff, J. 1996. *Saint Louis*, Paris: Gallinaud.

Lévi-Strauss, C. 1969. *The Elementary Structures of Kinship (Les Structures élémentaires de la Parenté)*, Boston: Beacon Press.

Mira, M.T., Alcaïs, A., Van Thuc, N., Thai, V.H., Huong, N.T., Ba, N.N., Verner, A., Hudson, T.J., Abel, L. and Schurr, E. 2003. 'Chromosome 6q25 is linked to susceptibility to leprosy in a Vietnamese population', *Nature genetics*, **33**, 412-415.

de Miramon, C. 1999. *Les 'donnés' au Moyen Âge. Une forme de vie religieuse laïque (v. 1180 – v. 1500)*, Paris: Le Cerf.

Moore, R.I. 2007. *The Formation of Persecuting Society. Authority and Deviance in Western Europe 950-1250*, Malden: Wiley.

Moore, R.I. 2012. *The War on Heresy: Faith and Power in Medieval Europe*, Cambridge: Belknap Press of Harvard University Press.

Nirenberg, D. 1996. *Communities of Violence. Persecution of Minorities in the Middle Ages*, Princeton: Princeton University Press.

Ortner, D.J. 2002. 'Observations on the pathogenesis of skeletal disease in leprosy', in M.E. Lewis, K. Manchester and C.A. Roberts (eds), *The past and present of leprosy. Archaeological, historical, palaeopathological and clinical approaches*, 73-77. Oxford: BAR Publishing.

Pastoureau, M. 1989. 'L'Église et la couleur, des origines à la Réforme', *Bibliothèque de l'École des Chartes*, **147**, 202-230.

Pattyn, S.R., Docks, P. and Cap, J.A. 1981. *La lèpre. Microbiologie, diagnostic, traitement et lutte. Manuel à l'usage du personnel médical et paramédical*, Paris: Masson.

Piponnier, F. and Mane, P. 1995. *Se vêtir au Moyen Âge*, Paris: A. Biro.

Pontal, O. (ed.) 1983. *Les statuts synodaux français du XIIIᵉ siècle, II: Les statuts de 1230 à 1260*, Paris: CTHS.

Ranque, B. 2008. 'La lèpre: un paradigme pour l'étude de la prédisposition génétique aux maladies infectieuses', *Médecine/Science*, **24(5)**, 491-497.

Rawcliffe, C. 2006. *Leprosy in Medieval England*, Woodbridge: Boydell Press.

Robertson Smith, W. 1889 (repr. 2005). *Lectures on the religion of the Semites. The Fundamental Institutions*, London: Adam and Charles Black.

Robertson, J.C. (ed.) 1875. *Materials for the History of Thomas Becket, Archbishop of Canterbury (Canonized by Pope Alexander III, A.D. 1173): Vol. I, William of Canterbury: Vita, passio et miracula S. Thomæ Cantuariensis archiepiscopi*, London: Longman.

Robertson, J.C. (ed.) 1876. *Materials for the History of Thomas Becket, Archbishop of Canterbury (Canonized by Pope Alexander III, A.D. 1173): Vol. II, Benedict of Peterborough, Passio sancti Thomæ Cantuariensis*, London: Longman.

Roch, J.L. 1989. 'Le jeu de l'aumône au Moyen Âge', *Annales. Économies, Sociétés, Civilisations*, **44(3)**, 505-528.

Sansarricq, H. (ed.) 1995. *La lèpre*, Paris: Ellipses.

Scubla, L. 1998. 'Fonction symbolique et fondement sacrificiel des sociétés humaines', *La Revue du* MAUSS, **12**, 41-65.

Sigal, P.A. 2001. 'Naissance et développement d'un vinage exceptionnel: l'eau de saint Thomas', *Cahiers de civilisation médiévale*, **44**, 35-44.

Sot, M. 1985. 'Mépris du monde et résistance des corps aux XIᵉ et XIIᵉ siècles', *Médiévales*, **8** 12-14.

Tarot, C. 2012. 'Les lyncheurs et le concombre ou de la définition de la religion quand même', in A. Caillé (ed), *Qu'est-ce que le religieux? Religion et politique*, 263-292. Paris: Revue du MAUSS.

Théry, J. 2003. '*Fama*: l'opinion publique comme preuve judiciaire. Aperçu sur la révolution médiévale de l'inquisitoire (XIIᵉ – XIVᵉ siècle)', in B. Lemesle (ed.), *La preuve en justice de l'Antiquité à nos jours*: 119-147. Rennes: Presses de Rennes.

Touati, F.O. 1991. 'Les léproseries aux XIIᵉ et XIIIᵉ siècles, des lieux de conversions?', in N. Bériou and F.O. Touati, *Voluntate Dei leprosus. Les lépreux entre conversion et exclusion aux XIIᵉ et XIIIᵉ siècles*, 2-32. Spoleto: Fondazione CISAM.

Touati, F.O. 1998. *Maladie et société au Moyen Âge. La lèpre, les lépreux et les léproseries dans la province ecclésiastique de Sens, jusqu'au milieu du XIVᵉ siècle*, Paris and Brussel: De Boeck.

Touati, F.O. 2000. 'Contagion and leprosy: myths, ideas and evolution in medieval minds and societies', in L. Conrad and D. Wujastyk (eds.), *Contagion: perspectives from Pre-modern Societies*, 179-201. London: Ashgate Publishing Limited.

Vauchez, A. 1993. 'Le tournant pastoral de l'Église en Occident', in A. Vauchez (ed), *Histoire du christianisme. Apogée de la chrétienté (1054-1274)* (Vol 5), 737-793. Paris: Desclée.

Vincent, C. 1988. *Des charités bien ordonnées. Les confréries normandes à la fin du XIIᵉ siècle, au début du XVIᵉ siècle*, Paris: Ecole Normale Superieure.

Vincent, C. 1991. 'Y a-t-il une mathématique du salut dans les diocèses du nord de la France à la veille de la Réforme?', *Revue de l'histoire de l'Église de France*, **77**, 137-149.

Vincent, C. 1994. *Les confréries médiévales dans le royaume de France, XIIIᵉ-XVᵉ siècle*, Paris: Editions Albin Michel.

Wilmotte, M. (ed.) 1927. *Chrétien de Troyes: Guillaume d'Angleterre. Roman du XIIᵉ siècle*, Paris: Champion.